Affonso Renato Meira

Abortion

Affonso Renato Meira

Abortion

Introduction and perspectives

ScienciaScripts

Imprint

Any brand names and product names mentioned in this book are subject to trademark, brand or patent protection and are trademarks or registered trademarks of their respective holders. The use of brand names, product names, common names, trade names, product descriptions etc. even without a particular marking in this work is in no way to be construed to mean that such names may be regarded as unrestricted in respect of trademark and brand protection legislation and could thus be used by anyone.

Cover image: Provided by the author

This book is a translation from the original published under ISBN 978-3-330-75417-1.

Publisher:
Sciencia Scripts
is a trademark of
Dodo Books Indian Ocean Ltd. and OmniScriptum S.R.L publishing group

120 High Road, East Finchley, London, N2 9ED, United Kingdom
Str. Armeneasca 28/1, office 1, Chisinau MD-2012, Republic of Moldova, Europe
Managing Directors: Ieva Konstantinova, Victoria Ursu
info@omniscriptum.com

Printed at: see last page
ISBN: 978-620-8-04616-3

**Dedicated to
Jo, Silvia,
Douglas,
Rodolpho, with
all my love.**

Preface

The preface to a book is a place reserved by the author for a name recognized for its value on the subject, or for a friend, to whom he wants to pay homage, to write it.

However, there are occasions when the plaintiff finds it difficult or embarrassing to make this request. And when the subject is controversial, there are different positions.

This is precisely what happens with the subject discussed in this work, all the more so because it is approached from different perspectives.

When it comes to abortion, one of two positions is taken: either you're for it, or you're against it.

This book brings to light the most varied positions, with approaches from a medical, cultural, historical, ethical, religious, social and legal point of view, often placed in isolation or sometimes in conjunction or relative, without imposing anything decisive.

With each point of view, you can find a name of recognized value and persuasiveness defending its idea, which is antagonistic to another that has the same recognition in society. The main purpose of this work is to offer the reader the possibility of discerning. This is also the reason why no positions are found that are openly for or against abortion.

Whether to invite a Minister of the Court or a Minister of a Church is a question that has no answer.

In this work there are many different statements defending or attacking this surgical act, without trying to highlight a definitive position, because it is really up to the woman and the doctor to decide on abortion. These are the people who, depending on the culture of the society in which they live, can have the freedom to perform it in a lawful, correct and safe way or hidden in the shadows, in an illicit, much more unsafe and incorrect way. However, who decides whether to allow or punish those who do it is society through prison or the church through sin.

In fact, not all religions consider abortion a violation of their dogmas, nor do all societies consider abortion a breach of their laws.

Perhaps these and other discrepancies that are revealed in this book to bring out the different perspectives on abortion, will make the reader understand and forgive why the preface was written by the author.

Summary

1 Introduction

The title of this article, "Introduction and Perspectives", is meant to reflect the intention of taking a broader approach, albeit at an introductory level, to a subject that has already been dealt with, without contradicting or discrediting it, but rather adding new information. Giving the title "Abortion: introduction and perspectives" to complement a work published under the title "Abortion: reflections" (17) in no way detracts from what has been done. The idea is to make it bigger, now with data from research and surveys that have already been published, decisions made by the courts and a historical approach that brings to mind what other cultures have to say on the subject.

In addition, passages from different times that show the importance of the subject are presented as necessary perspectives for concluding on this controversial subject. The prelude to man on earth; the emergence of abortion and its history; the beginning of life; life being sacred and having to be lived without quality; the influence of religions and legislations; the difference in different cultures; are all aspects that are addressed and must be analyzed, among others, in order to be able to discern. Some of the research carried out in the book can provide a firmer basis for the configurations drawn up.

The presence of this data enriches and strengthens the statements previously made, guaranteeing a publicized position on a relevant social fact such as abortion.

In any case, it cannot be a continuation, a revision or a contradiction. It is more than anything a complement. If there is a sin in this elaboration, it lies in the desire to go beyond the level of an article that was published as an editorial in a journal, the most prestigious in the field in Brazil, even reaching international interest. Once this level has been reached, there is the possibility that these prospects could be realized in the form of a book. This is a valid and desired quest.

It's not a pretension to be pursued at any cost or by disfiguring the original ideas. If the edition can't be found, the value of continuing a work that has earned praise can't be disfigured in any way, because the intention of a piece of writing is to disseminate the thoughts and values of the author. It is not the presentation, which can vary from a manuscript to a rich edition on the finest cover and paper, that constitutes the quality of the writing. The quality of the writing reflects the validity of the subject and of the person who wrote it.

Abortion is one of the most controversial issues in the medical field. The problem of abortion is a clear example both of the difficulty of establishing social dialogues in the face of differing moral positions and of the obstacle in creating an independent academic discourse Addressing it has an established meaning, being for or against it. Even if society as a whole does not have a greater commitment to enforcing a position and accepts existing legal positions with little discussion, it is necessary to deal with the religious, social and ethical aspects in which the country's culture is involved.

Some facts are quite clear about the woman and the doctor, who are the characters in this medical action and who are often prevented or punished by society when they decide to have an abortion.

It should be borne in mind that: those who want a pregnancy do not want an abortion; those who want an abortion cannot have or do not want a child; medicine is not against abortion; neither the woman nor the doctor is obliged to have an abortion; it is society that decides whether or not to have an abortion.

In modern societies where medicine is centered on experiments and research derived from scientific knowledge, it is often difficult for doctors to complete their actions in a way that is desirable. This is because in these societies the knowledge of the people, transcribed and incorporated into cultures, comes from different sources.

There are different ways of acquiring knowledge and absorbing it into the culture of societies. This is also the case in the same society, where different strata have different knowledge. This depends on the composition of these layers due to education, economic power, religious belief, ethics, racial composition and many other less preponderant factors. However, there are four main ways in which this knowledge can be established as a solid foundation: the philosophical, which arises from disputes during discussions; the empirical, which is the product of observations focused from different angles; the analogical, which comes from comparisons of the same or different facts and objects; and finally the scientific, which is produced by research and experiments that vary widely.

These paths are enveloped by these various factors and by the environment so that they merge into the culture of the population and diversify across the layers of society. In this way, aspects of health come to be analyzed from various angles. The different angles that translate into a new perspective are: the vacillating, indecisive, perplexed biological thought - life;
legal thinking: precise, concise, fair - texts, codes and laws;
ethical thinking: first causes, customs - virtue;
religious thought: dogmas, the supernatural - the church;
bioethical thinking: holistic, comprehensive - the question.

Whereas in pagan societies the solution to health problems is sought by the peasant, who solves them within his capacity and competence by seeking knowledge obtained through tradition and observation; in modern societies the solution to health issues is brought to doctors or other professionals linked to medical studies, whose knowledge, although in part it may be the product of observation and comparison, is based on research and experiments, in other words, on the scientific method.

There is only one way to obtain the scientific knowledge that guides doctors in their work, and that is to seek it out at a medical school and graduate as a doctor.

Doctor and patient are in the position of increasingly wanting the latest technology in care and treatment, matching the doctor's interests, whether financial, ethical or scientific, with those of the patient (12).

On many occasions, the doctor and his client, who have different opinions, disagree on whether to carry out a proposed medical act. In today's societies, it is considered an ethical obligation for the doctor to respect the patient's autonomy of decision.

Part of an already elaborate writing allows for a greater understanding of the relationship between the doctor and the client:

After the Second World War ended in 1945, there was a new view of the world arising from the victory of the Allied countries against the Axis countries. World public opinion saw the victory of democracy over dictatorship.

There was an increase in medicine with the discovery of antibiotics, the use of vaccines and the development of technology allowing for more aggressive surgeries. At the same time, there was concern about the social aspects of health, which originated with Winslow's 1925 conceptualization of public health:

The science and art of preventing disease, prolonging life, promoting health and physical and mental efficiency, through the organized efforts of the community for: the sanitation of the environment - the control of transmissible diseases - the education of the person in principles of personal hygiene - the organization of medical and nursing services - the early diagnosis and treatment of diseases - the development of social machinery.

The United Nations Organization promulgated the Declaration of Human Rights with the concern of protecting individuals in 1948.

Assembly of the World Health Association of the World Health Organization in 1949 promulgated an International Code of Ethics.

The same World Health Organization, indicating a trend, at its 1951 Assembly, conceptualized health as *"a state of perfect physical, mental and social well-being and not merely the absence of disease or infirmity. "*.

Concern about racial integration and human rights movements were issues of interest to American society in the 1960s. Dorothy Height, president of the National Council of Negro Women, helped Martin Luther King to orchestrate the struggle for black civil rights. The sad Tuskegee study, carried out on blacks in Alabama to study the evolution of syphilis, was becoming known not only to those involved in health issues, but also to society as a whole.

American institutions, such as the Milbank Memorial Fund, which from 1962 promoted a five-year program that awarded fellowships to professors of health sciences who related to social sciences in the three Americas, demonstrated a direction in considering the importance of society's involvement with aspects of medical care, as well as with the teaching of health sciences.

In 1964, the World Medical Association drew up principles governing the behavior of researchers in experiments on the human species, known as the Declaration of Helsinki. Two years later, other international covenants were adopted by the United Nations General Assembly: the International Covenant on Civil and Political Rights and the International Covenant on Economic, Social and Cultural Rights.

Increased population growth was a cause for concern. Malthus resurfaced. The use of contraceptive pills was spreading. The debate about the ethical aspects of using the intrauterine device grew. In 1968, the Ford Foundation and the Population Council awarded Daniel Callahan a grant to study the ethical implications of birth control and family planning.

On the other hand, the development of medicine, such as transplants and the still remote possibility of assisted human reproduction, gave those who considered life to be sacred a sense of insecurity about what was happening in the health sector.

American society was undergoing a transformation in relation to the racial problem with a predominance of whites, Anglo-Saxons and Protestants who were beginning to lose strength. In this society, medicine was characterized by being ethnocentric, with the doctor exercising a defensive clinic, without concern for the patient's consent.

With these characteristics, the doctor, having received little training in ethics, defended himself against the establishment of health care groups and worried about his training as a specialist, which varied from state to state.

It was in this environment that an article written by Henry Beecher, Professor of Anesthesiology at Harvard Medical School, appeared in the June 1966 issue of the England Journal of Medicine, a prestigious medical journal published in Massachusetts, USA, under the title "Ethics in Clinical Research". In this article, which had not previously been accepted for publication in the Journal of the American Medical Association, the author listed twenty-two studies with unquestionable attitudes in which medical ethics were not respected.

The revelation of Beecher's article provoked countless comments and reflections, not only among health professionals but also among society in general, which was following experiments that were aggressive to human beings - such as the heart transplant carried out in 1967.

The teaching of ethics in medical schools in the United States was more intense in those with a Catholic religious orientation and it was in these schools that Beecher's work had an intense repercussion, leading the others to come under pressure, including from doctors and their students, to start discussing the ethical aspects of medicine.

This concern about how health, life and death were understood by those in society who were given the go-ahead to take care of them led American scholars such as Daniel Callahan, Willard Gayling, James Drane, Andre Hellegers, Van Rensselaer Potter and others to discuss and meditate on events relating to health, life and death. The reflections coming from the scholars were complemented by the different layers of society that brought to light the knowledge obtained by the different ways of getting to know.

In the Spring 1969 issue of the journal Daedolus, a paper by 6 doctors, 5 lawyers, 1 anthropologist, 1 sociologist, 1 philosopher, and 1 psychiatrist was published under the title "Ethical Aspects of Experiments with Human Subjects", addressing this concern in American society. The right of postulants became popular in American society in the 1970s. The health aspects of life and death became everyone's business.

It was from this mixture of means for the search for truth and virtue that the thought of what came to be called bioethics emerged. The name bioethics came about because in January 1971, Van Rensselaer Potter, an American oncologist, published a work dealing with aspects of health and the environment, entitled "Bioethics: the bridge to the future".

In the middle of the same year, Andre Hellegers, a Dutch-born obstetrician and gynecologist who emigrated to the United States in 1952 at the age of 27, founded the

"Joseph and Rose Kennedy Institute for Human Reproduction and Bioethics" at Georgetown University. This coincidence led to the spread of this term to name these meditations. The term bioethics had already been coined by Fritz Lahar in a publication in 1927, which, however, had no repercussions.

In any case, the neologism was discussed and accepted. Interpreted differently, by different and debatable visions of what was correct, the use of the term became irreversible.

Bioethics, Meira's concept expressed in 2000:

"comprises the study, analysis, reflection and thought that seek the conduct of the person in relation to health, life and death, according to the social ideal, based on the reasonableness of scientific knowledge, the emotions of people and the values of culture."

The first group of professors involved in these reflections at the Kennedy Institute of Bioethics was made up of Walters Le Roy from Theology; Thomaz Beauchamps from Philosophy; James Childress from Religious Studies; Edmund Pellegrino from Medicine and Robert Veatch from Medical Ethics. This union of scholars from different areas, but with the same objective of studying the aspects of health in its broadest approach, shows from the outset the transdisciplinary nature of the subject.

Two of these forerunners published a book "Beauchamp and Childress in 1984, in which they presented four principles to which doctors and other health professionals should adhere regardless of priority". Autonomy, beneficence, non-maleficence and justice.

Autonomy refers to the patient, while beneficence, non-maleficence and justice refer to the doctor's relationship with the patient.

Autonomy means the patient's right to be correctly informed about their health situation and the treatment offered by the doctor, as well as the possibilities of the expected end results, and to have the right to accept it or not. Autonomy is self-government, the ability to decide what you think is good and what is best for you. Beneficence means that the doctor should only do what is best for the patient, non-maleficence means not doing anything that could harm the patient and justice means treating everyone equally without discrimination.

Those who oppose abortion deny the woman's right to abortion because they claim that the fetus, once delivered, is another person. These people, instead of accepting autonomy, consider that this is a decision that illustrates heteronomy.

Bioethics was brought to Brazil by Meira, as Mainetti points out in "The Development of Bioethics in Latin America." *"In Sao Paulo, Brazil, bioethics was introduced by Affonso Renato Meira of the Oscar Freire Institute of the Faculty of Medicine of the University of Sao Paulo in 1990. "* began to be discussed in certain medical education centers in Brazil.(15).

After a critical reception, the principles proposed by Beauchamp and Childress were included in the principles of Brazilian medical ethics and are now included not only in treaties, but also in the codes that cover the subject.

In the Code of Medical Ethics (3), the autonomy of the patient is preserved in the Fundamental Principles XXI -

"In the process of making professional decisions, in accordance with the dictates of their conscience and the provisions of the law, doctors will accept their patients' choices regarding the diagnostic and therapeutic procedures they express, provided that they are appropriate to the case and scientifically recognized."

Chapter IV of the Code of Medical Ethics (3), which deals with human rights, states in Art. 22 that a doctor may not:

"Failing to obtain the consent of the patient or their legal representative after explaining the procedure to them, except in cases of imminent risk of death."

Further on in Chapter V Relations with Patients and Relatives, Article 31 states that a doctor is forbidden:

"Disrespecting the right of the patient or their legal representative to freely decide on the execution of diagnostic or therapeutic practices except in the case of imminent risk of death"

If the patient does not accept what the doctor considers should be done to treat the patient, the doctor is not obliged to accept the patient's decision. The Code of Medical Ethics (3) states: Art. 36.§1.

"In the event of events which, in their judgment, jeopardize the good relationship with the patient or full professional performance, the doctor has the right to resign from the service provided that they give prior notice to the patient or their legal representative, ensuring continuity of care and providing all the necessary information to the doctor who will succeed them."

What is debatable is who decides, or who approves the decision made by the doctor. When there is nothing to discuss, the doctor explains his decision and the patient accepts it. The interpretation to be sought is that when the doctor, in his paternalistic action, does not accept the patient's rejection, the patient in turn does not agree with the doctor's decision. Both parties - the doctor and the client - have vulnerable points in this relationship.

What is desirable in this relationship is sometimes far from being achieved. And society as a whole is perhaps the most responsible, and the most damaged, because even with the will to solve this dilemma, it has so far failed to achieve this goal.

In bringing up ethics as a reason for the doctor's behavior, it's important to clarify a confusion often made between ethics and morality.

These words differ in their origin, but have the same meaning. Etica from the

Greek *ethike* and moral from the Latin mos, *moris,* are translated into Portuguese as customs. Some scholars call the ideal order for human activities moral and the social order actually established by custom and practice, ethical. Others invert these denominations, calling the ideal order ethics and the order established by uses and customs morals. In addition to these orders, we must also remember the individual ethics or morals that reveal a person's conscience.

The "ought to be" is the imperative of ideal ethics or morality. "How to do it" is the determinant of social ethics or morality. "What I think I should do" is the result of individual ethics or morality. Many people don't differentiate between the use of these terms, and so the term ethics is used here for the sake of choice.

Ethics as a view of the world, in one era, differs from past and/or future times, and history demonstrates this fact. However, the validity of ethics in the present time is so strong that it is often difficult to understand its changes.

Abortion is one of the aspects of the practice of medicine which, because of its religious and ethical aspects, as well as its legal and ethnic aspects, has the greatest difficulty in producing a unity of opinion in different societies. Thus, in some societies abortion is totally forbidden, in others it is totally allowed, and between these extremes there are societies that allow it with greater or lesser restrictions.

In the same way that societies, people of different faiths, ethnicities and backgrounds differ in their understanding and acceptance or disapproval of a medical procedure.

This divergence often occurs between the doctor and his patient, especially when other variables from non-scientific knowledge interfere. This is the case with abortion.

2 Abortion

Abortion refers to the biological event of the expulsion of a dead fetus from the body of a woman or female animal, the product of which is known as abortion. So don't confuse abortion as the product of the procedure of its expulsion from the woman's body - which constitutes abortion - as is the case in the Brazilian Penal Code (3), which literally penalizes abortion, but with the aim of punishing those who produce abortion. The term abortion in current Portuguese also means failure. Like the verb abortar, it means to stop, to fail.

The fetus can come out of the pregnant woman's uterus naturally or by provocation before the pregnancy cycle is completed. Naturally occurring abortion is considered an event that should only be recorded, attended to and cared for when a new pregnancy occurs. Induced abortion can be performed using medication or by surgery. An abortion performed after taking medication can be confused with a naturally occurring abortion.

From a medical point of view, abortion should only be performed by a doctor with full rights and knowledge, with the woman's consent, without religious, ethical or legal obstacles and preferably during the first twelve weeks of pregnancy. The importance of this procedure has led the World Health Organization to publish a book on safe abortion, which is now in its second edition. (20) Termination of pregnancy, when carried out under the right conditions with adequate assistance, is a safe process.

Medical abortion

Despite the restrictions on abortion in Brazil, the country's Federal Council of Medicine has established ethical standards for doctors to use Emergency Contraception, which has the characteristics of a medical abortion. One aspect of this resolution is noteworthy. This medication, commonly known as the "morning-after pill", was banned from being imported and prescribed in Brazil for around ten years. This ban was always supported by religious groups and never challenged by medical institutions or associations. The Resolution (4) that now allows the use of this medication dates from 2006 and is currently in force:

CFM Resolution No. 1811 of December 14, 2006.
Diario Oficial da Uniao, Poder Executivo, Brasilia, DF January 17, 2007.
The Federal Council of Medicine, using the powers conferred by Law No. 3.268 of September 30, 1957, as amended by Law No. 11.000 of December 15, 2004, regulated by Decree No. 44.045 of July 19, 1958, and.

WHEREAS reproductive rights are based on the principles of human dignity and promote the exercise of responsible parenthood;

WHEREAS it is the State's responsibility to provide educational, scientific and material resources for the exercise of this right, and any coercive action by public or private entities is prohibited;

WHEREAS in Brazil there is a significant number of women exposed to unwanted pregnancies, either through the non-use or inadequate use of contraceptive methods;

WHEREAS the groups most affected are adolescents and young adults, who often begin sexual activity before contraception.

WHEREAS preventing unwanted pregnancies is a good example of responsible sexuality, and such pregnancies can lead to psychic and social costs that are sometimes irreversible;

WHEREAS the practice of dual protection - recommended by the World Health Organization, the Ministry of Health, the Brazilian Federation of Gynecology and Obstetrics Societies and the Brazilian Society of Pediatrics, seeks to instill the use of male or female condoms, concomitant with another contraceptive method, including Emergency Contraception;

WHEREAS emergency contraception can be used at any stage of reproductive life and phase of the menstrual cycle to prevent pregnancy and, in the event of fertilization, there will be no interruption of the gestational process;

WHEREAS the aim of emergency contraception is to prevent pregnancy and even in the rare case of failure the method does not cause damage to the progress of the pregnancy;

WHEREAS Emergency Contraception can contribute to reducing unwanted pregnancies and induced abortions;

WHEREAS, finally, the decision taken at the plenary session held on December 14, 2006,

RESOLVE:

Art. 1 Accept Emergency Contraception as an alternative method for preventing pregnancy, as it does not cause harm or interrupt pregnancy.

Art. 2 - It is the doctor's responsibility to prescribe Emergency Contraception as a preventive measure, in order to interfere with the negative impact of unplanned pregnancy and its consequences on Public Health, particularly reproductive health.

Art. 3 - For the practice of Emergency Contraception, the methods currently in use or which may be developed, accepted by the scientific community and which comply with Brazilian legislation, i.e. which are not abortifacients, may be used.

Art. 4 Emergency contraception can be used at all stages of reproductive life.

Art. 5 All provisions to the contrary are hereby repealed.

Art. 6 This resolution shall enter into force on the date of its publication.

Brasilia-DF, December 14, 2006.

EDSON DE OLIVEIRA ANDRADE
President of the Council

Livia Barros Gargao Council Secretary

Because this method has always been criticized and considered abortifacient by many, it needed a lot of justification to be allowed through a resolution by the Brazilian Federal Council of Medicine. Everything from the World Health Organization to the Brazilian Society of Pediatrics was consulted to justify the use of this method.

Marcelo Zugaib, Professor and Head of the Department of Gynecology and Obstetrics at the University of Sao Paulo Medical School, is in favor of the Federal Council of Medicine's resolution on Emergency Contraception. However, he points out that the so-called morning-after pill "is an abortifacient and that the pregnant woman should be informed of this in order to make a decision." (9).

No reference to institutions concerned with ethics in relation to health, and not even an explanation of what is considered to be established as Emergency Contraception. Which drug or drugs are allowed. It's a dubious resolution.

There is no such thing as pogao tea or any herb that is effective in producing abortion.

The World Health Organization (20) recommends that mefepristone 200 mg should always be used orally and that misoprostol should be indicated 1 to 2 days later. Depending on whether it's vaginal, buccal, sublingual or oral, the dose of misoprostol is 8oo mg.

Medical abortion should be started as soon as possible after sexual intercourse.

Surgical abortion

Surgical abortion is always provoked or induced for medical or legal reasons. For this reason, surgical abortion should be performed, if possible, before the 12th week of pregnancy in an aseptic environment such as an operating room, with all the care required for a correct procedure. In addition to being examined for the possibility of taking pre-anesthetic medication and the conditions for surgery, the patient needs to be admitted to hospital and undergo anesthesia. Depending on the woman's condition, anesthesia can be obtained by airway, intravenous or spinal anesthesia. It is therefore a hospital procedure. The fetus is removed by vacuum aspiration, intrauterine, at a maximum of 12 to 14 weeks of the patient's gestation. The method of dilation and curettage, if still practiced, should be replaced by vacuum aspiration. (20) The use of the dilatation and curettage method has led to abortion being referred to as curettage in Brazil.

Other techniques are used for abortion. These include the cutting method, which is used at the beginning of pregnancy. A scraper is inserted into the woman's uterus to separate the fetus and cut it into pieces, which produces very intense bleeding. (9) Another way of producing abortion is by injecting saline directly into the fetus, which loses its vital functions within an hour. (10)

In the face of legislation in countries where there are few opportunities to perform this operation without incurring a penalty, it is often carried out in far from ideal conditions. And abortion performed in precarious conditions is far from what is lawful. The Federal Council of Medicine, faced with the Brazilian Supreme Court's decision that abortion performed on women with anencephalic fetuses does not constitute a crime, issued the following resolution:

    CFM Resolution 1.989/2012 published in the D.O.U.
    of May 14, 2012,Segao I,p.308 and 309

Provides for the diagnosis of anencephaly for the therapeutic anticipation of childbirth and other measures.

THE FEDERAL COUNCIL OF MEDICINE, using the powers conferred by Law No. 3.268, of September 30, 1957, amended by Law No. 11.000, of December 15, 2004, regulated by Decree No. 44.045, of July 19, 1955,and

CONSIDERING the Code of Medical Ethics (CFM Resolution No. 1931/09, published in the Official Gazette of September 24, 2009, Section I, p. 90, republished in the Official Gazette of October 13, 2009, Section I, p.173);

WHEREAS the Federal Supreme Court upheld the Argument for Non-Compliance with Fundamental Precept No. 54, of June 17, 2004 (ADPF-54), and declared the constitutionality of the therapeutic anticipation of childbirth in cases of anencephalic fetus, which does not characterize the abortion typified in articles 124, 126 and 128 (items I and II) of the Penal Code, nor is it to be confused with it;

WHEREAS the factual premise of this judgment is the unequivocal medical diagnosis of anencephaly;

WHEREAS it is up to the Federal Council of Medicine to define the criteria for diagnosing anencephaly;

WHEREAS the diagnosis of anencephaly is made by ultrasound examination;

WHEREAS it is the exclusive competence of the doctor to carry out and interpret the ultrasound examination on human beings, as well as to issue the respective report, in accordance with the following terms

of CFMn Resolution⁰ 1.361/92, of December 9, 1992 (Published in the D.O. U. of December 14, 1992, Section I, p. 17.186);

WHEREAS the Medical Councils are, at the same time, judges and disciplinarians of the medical profession, and it is up to them to watch over and work, with all the means at their disposal, for the prestige and good reputation of the profession and for the perfect ethical performance of the professionals who practice medicine legally;

WHEREAS the goal of all medical care is the health of the human being, for whose benefit they must act with the utmost care and to the best of their professional ability;

CONSIDERING article 10, item III of the Federal Constitution, which chose the principle of the dignity of the human person as one of the foundations of the Federative Republic of Brazil;

WHEREAS article 50, III of the Federal Constitution states that no one shall be subjected to torture or inhuman or degrading treatment;

WHEREAS it is the doctor's responsibility to ensure the well-being of patients;

CONSIDERING the contents of the explanatory memorandum accompanying this resolution;

WHEREAS, finally, the decision taken at the plenary session of the Federal Council of Medicine held on May 10, 2012,

RESOLVE:

Art. 10

In the event of an unequivocal diagnosis of anencephaly, the doctor may terminate the pregnancy at the request of the pregnant woman, regardless of state authorization.

Art. 2º
The diagnosis of anencephaly is made by an ultrasound scan carried out from the 12thª (twelfth) week of pregnancy onwards:
I- -two photographs, identified and dated: one showing the face of the fetus in a sagittal position; the other showing the cephalic pole in cross-section, demonstrating the absence of the skullcap and identifiable brain parenchyma;
II- -a report signed by two doctors who are qualified to make this diagnosis.

Art. 3º
Once the diagnosis of anencephaly has been made, the doctor must provide the pregnant woman with all the clarifications requested, guaranteeing her the right to decide freely on the course of action to be adopted, without imposing his authority to induce her to make any decision or to limit her in what she decides.
§Paragraph 1 - It is the pregnant woman's right to request a medical panel or to seek another opinion on the diagnosis.
§Paragraph 2: In the event of a diagnosis of anencephaly, the pregnant woman has the right to:
I - maintain the pregnancy;
II - terminate the pregnancy immediately, regardless of the length of the pregnancy, or postpone the decision until another time.
§Paragraph 3 - Whatever the pregnant woman's decision, the doctor must inform her of the consequences, including the risks arising from or associated with each.
§Paragraph 4 - If the pregnant woman chooses to continue with the pregnancy, she shall be guaranteed prenatal medical care commensurate with the diagnosis.
§Paragraph 5: Both the pregnant woman who chooses to maintain her pregnancy and the one who chooses to terminate it will receive, if they so wish, assistance from a multi-professional team in the places where it is available.
§Paragraph 6. Therapeutic anticipation of childbirth may only be carried out in a hospital that has adequate facilities for the treatment of possible complications inherent in the respective procedures.

Art. 4
Minutes shall be drawn up of the therapeutic anticipation of childbirth, which shall include the consent of the pregnant woman and/or, where appropriate, her legal representative. The minutes, photographs and report of the examination referred to in Article 2 of this resolution shall be included in the patient's medical record.

Art. 5
Once the therapeutic anticipation of childbirth has been carried out, the doctor must inform the patient of the risks of recurrence of the anencephaly and refer her to family planning programs with contraception assistance, as long as this is necessary, and

preconception, when it is freely desired, always guaranteeing the woman's right to choose.
Sole paragraph.
The patient should be explicitly informed that preconception care is aimed at reducing the recurrence of anencephaly.

Art. 6
This resolution enters into force on the date of its publication.

Brasilia
DF, May 10, 2012
CARLOS VITAL TAVARES CORREA LIMA
President-in-Office
HENRIQUE BATISTA E SILVA
General secretary

Illicit abortion

Abortion is either accepted or penalized due to the different tendencies of different societies with different ethnicities and cultures.
In countries with a Catholic majority, acceptance is limited to special situations, as is the case in South America. In Europe there is a divergence between Latin and other nations. In the United States of America, there are differences in legal procedures between states. What does happen, however, is that when abortion is not accepted by the law, it is still sought by women for a variety of reasons. It is sought illegally and carried out without the knowledge of family and friends. The woman often finds herself alone or accompanied by an accomplice. Ethically concerned hospitals and doctors who are concerned about the law do not perform them.

These abortions are carried out by doctors who are unconcerned about ethics and legislation in clinics or in their offices. Midwives or curious women carry out this type of intervention under worse conditions. Often, the pregnant woman is tied up with her legs spread and curetted without anesthesia. If it's impossible to find someone to carry out the abortion, on other occasions it's carried out by the woman herself, inserting objects into the vaginal cavity or using oral, venous or local drugs. She doesn't bother with anything other than expelling the fetus from her uterus.

3 Cultural and historical aspects.

History should not be seen as a mere cycle of life, which reports nothing more than the passage of time, but rather as a way of gaining an understanding of why things happened.

By bringing up historical aspects of abortion over time, it is necessary to analyze this passage, which in the same society also leads to changes in these cultures. Although the importance of women's education will be analyzed when trying to estimate the number of abortions performed, on this occasion the term culture will be used as it is used in the social sciences, especially in cultural anthropology. To do this, we will look to Edward Taylor for a conceptualization of culture: "it is the whole complex which includes beliefs, arts, morals, law, customs as well as all the abilities and habits acquired by man as a member of a society." (12). In anthropological terms, culture is considered to be a people's way of thinking, feeling and acting. This includes communication, knowledge, beliefs, skills, feelings, tastes, organization, production and everything else that society does to satisfy itself.

Culture has two levels of standards: an ideal standard and a practical or real level of culture. Kluckhohn (12) calls the ideal standard the one that determines what to do and the practical standard the one that shows the behavior adopted. In addition to these other aspects are found:

1. culture is a universal phenomenon, all human societies are guided by some form of culture. Although it is possible to find universal aspects in all cultures, local or regional manifestations are diverse, showing that each society is governed by the values of its own culture;

2. culture fills and determines action in the lives of all human beings, but it does so unconsciously;

3. Culture is both stable and dynamic. It is static in order to maintain its values and dynamic in order to allow these values to change.

When dealing with the narrative of events that take place over time, it won't be possible to understand them unless we look at the places and societies where they took place. When looking for historical data, the cultural aspects of the different eras or places will undoubtedly come together and involve them. Therefore, without worrying about differentiating these areas, which is not the aim of this book, they have been included together without prejudice to the goal to be achieved, which is the presence of abortion in different eras and cultures.

There is no doubt that the role played by women in society varies according to the different cultures found around the world. In different societies, culture reserves a different position, role and behavior for women. While in Western societies the role and position of women includes politics, with women being able to reach or compete for the highest office in the nation's leadership allowed by legislation, as is or was the case in Argentina, Germany, Chile, France, Brazil, England, and the United States of North America, to name but a few, in other Eastern countries women are not allowed to stay with their husbands or their husband's friends, nor are they forbidden to go to beaches wearing swimsuits. Islamic countries require women to cover their faces with veils,

The position of abortion in these societies varies at different times, just as women's behavior varies according to what is imposed on them by the culture of society.

Among the many events that concern health professionals, abortion stands out because of the difficulty in presenting appropriate measures to minimize its effects on the population. The problem of abortion presents a difficulty in promoting dialog, since there are contradictory opinions. In different societies, there are ideal values in relation to abortion, in other words, that it should be carried out under the necessary conditions from a health point of view and always in accordance with ethical and legal precepts. However, the pattern of behavior shows that this ideal standard has often not been reached and abortion is carried out in violation of health precepts, ethics and the law.

If you look back in history for references to abortion, you'll find that the Hebrews had a code that punished those who performed abortions, even with the death penalty. (14) In Greek mythology, you'll find a quote from Aristotle, who was initially opposed to abortion and then agreed to it as long as the embryo was lifeless. Hippocrates - the father of medicine - in fact the forerunner of medical ethics, was the author of an oath that doctors must follow, in which the practice of abortion is forbidden. Hippocrates' oath, taken before Christ, states that "I will not give an abortifacient substance to any woman". (15) In the Code of Hammurabi, abortion is also punishable. In Sparta, abortion was forbidden because of the need for men to take charge of internal security and to form armies to intervene in times of war.

The question of abortion became a burning issue when St. Augustine spoke out on the subject, and then St. Thomas Aquinas, who differentiated between the formed and the unformed fetus. (14) In the Roman Empire, the question of abortion was also taken up.

From the eighteenth century onwards, despite the little interest abortion caused in societies, its practice was frowned upon, mainly because scientific knowledge had laid new foundations in the seventeenth and eighteenth centuries, leading to the fetus being recognized as an autonomous entity and religious affirmations being echoed in legislation.

With the French Revolution and the emergence of new nations, wars, plagues and geographical discoveries, new changes took place in the Western world: the population increase decreased, while the need to maintain a larger army increased. Men's lives became more valuable and motherhood a patriotic activity. (24)

In the nineteenth century, the idea of a large family led governments to protect the birth rate for eminent political and ideological reasons. After the Second World War, scientific knowledge revealed techniques and methods that allowed people to live longer. Even so, countries like France, Germany and Spain took more restrictive measures against abortion.

From the nineteen sixties onwards, a series of demonstrations in favor of abortion led governments to become concerned about these movements generated by women

With the development of scientific knowledge from the end of the 1970s, with new artificial fertilization techniques, and with concerns about population growth, one direction of scientific light took the path of hindering this advance. Thus, methods, techniques, uses and even beliefs to avoid pregnancy and birth were recalled.

In the United States of America, the guiding country of scientific education for less developed countries, there were movements for abortion not to be penalized, just as in Europe.

From 1996 to 2009, 47 countries of the World Health Organization passed more liberal abortion legislation, as opposed to 11 that tightened it. (2)

Groups in favor of abortion tried to justify it with allegations about cases in which pregnancy risked the health of the pregnant woman.

Pope John Paul II in the Vatican called on his followers not to subject themselves to abortion, the purpose of which was to affect a living being that was the product of conception.(**)

In Brazil, during this period and until today, the legislation has remained the same despite movements in favor of liberalization. (3) However, many abortions are carried out because the woman's life is at risk. The term "life-threatening" is much less restricted than "there is no other means of saving life". In fact, according to Gandra Martins (9), medical progress has reached such a level that there are practically no other means of saving a pregnant woman's life than abortion. (9)

The Regional Councils of Medicine at the 1st National Meeting of Medical Councils in 2013 (6) agreed that the Reform of the Penal Code, which was awaiting a vote, should rule out the illegality of terminating a pregnancy in one of the following situations:

a) when "there is a risk to the life or health of the pregnant woman; "

b) if "the pregnancy is the result of a violation of sexual dignity, or the non-

consensual use of assisted reproductive technology; "

c) if "anencephaly is proven or when the fetus suffers from serious and incurable

anomalies that make independent life impossible, in both cases attested by two

doctors;" and

d) if "by the will of the pregnant woman until the 12th week of pregnancy".[a]

From an ethical point of view, a majority of the meeting decided that the limits excluding the illegality of abortion laid down in the 1940 Penal Code, which had been respected by medical organizations, were inconsistent with humanistic and humanitarian commitments, paradoxical to social responsibility and the international treaties signed by the Brazilian government. (6)

In other countries, depending on culture, religiosity and legal aspects, there are different ways of approaching abortion.

Portugal has legalized abortion up to the 10th week of pregnancy. (9)

In Spain, abortion has been permitted since 1985 in cases of rape, fetal malformation and risk to the life or health of the pregnant woman. (9)

In Mexico, abortion is allowed up to the 12th week in the country's capital, but the situation is ambiguous in several states. (2)

In Uruguay, the bill was approved by the National Congress, but was vetoed by then President Tabare Vazquez. (2)

Colombia allowed abortion only in cases of rape and maternal risk or fetal malformation. Until then, abortion was forbidden. (2)

Nicaragua and the Dominican Republic have banned abortion. (2)

Since 1997, El Salvador has banned all types of abortion. (2) In this country, a woman who has a spontaneous abortion may be punished with the loss of her life if she cannot prove that the process was uninterrupted.

Argentina, Ecuador, Iraq and Japan have also tightened legislation restricting the practice of abortion. (2)

In Sweden, abortion is and has been unrestricted if performed up to the eighteenth week of pregnancy. (9)

The Netherlands was one of the first countries to allow abortion. There, abortion is free until the 22nd week of pregnancy (9).

Finland, one of the richest countries in the world, allows abortion up to the twelfth week of pregnancy if there are social reasons for doing so. (9)

In Germany, the law stipulates that a woman who wishes to undergo an abortion permitted by current legislation must have it approved by private doctors recognized by the government. In Bavaria, a law was passed prohibiting doctors from receiving more than 25% of their income from abortion. The German Constitutional Court declared this law unconstitutional because it endangered the health of the woman, who, unable to find a doctor who could perform the abortion in Germany, would seek it outside the country. (9)

Since 1983, abortion in Turkey has been permitted up to the 10th week of pregnancy. The decision to have an abortion is made by the woman who wishes to have it.

In Israel, abortion is permitted when there is a psychological or physical risk to the woman, in cases of fetal malformation, and also for humanitarian reasons. (24)

In Canada, abortion is legal. In Canada, there is legislation that allows nurses not to be forced to participate in abortions on the grounds of conscientious objection. (9) This position of claiming a reason of conscience must be analyzed very carefully, because otherwise anyone who is punished can claim to have acted out of conscience in order to escape the penalty.

In India, although Hinduism classifies abortion as an abominable act, in practice India has partially allowed abortion since 1971. However, the use of abortion as a form of child sex selection led the government to take action in 1994 against this particular practice. (**) Abortion is guaranteed in the following cases:

1. *The woman has a serious illness and the pregnancy could put her life at risk.*
2. *When a woman's physical or mental health is at risk during pregnancy,*
3. *When the fetus is at risk of being born with a physical or mental anomaly.*
4. *If the pregnant woman contracts rubeola during the first three months of pregnancy.*
5. *If the woman has previously given birth to children with congenital anomalies.*
6. *If the fetus has a blood disorder.*
7. *If the fetus has been exposed to radiation.*
8. *If the pregnancy is the result of rape.*
9. *If the pregnant woman's socio-economic situation hinders her pregnancy.*
10. *If the contraceptive has failed.*

If you have a second child or an unauthorized pregnancy in China, you will be forced to have an abortion. (**)

In Russia, abortion is legal up to 12^a weeks of pregnancy. In 1920, Russia became the first country in the world to allow abortion under all circumstances. However, over the course of the **twentieth century,** legislation on abortion in the country changed, and it was banned again in 1936, until 1954. According to data from the United Nations Organization, Russia has the highest number of abortions per woman of childbearing age in the world, between fifteen and forty-four, with around 1.3 million abortions (absolute number) carried out per year, which is equivalent to 53.7 abortions for every 1,000 women. (**)

Italian legislation before 1978 made it a crime to voluntarily terminate a pregnancy, but with the implementation of **Law 194 of** that year, voluntary abortion was decriminalized and can be performed up to the third month of pregnancy in Italian public hospitals, and in the 4th or 5th month in cases of a therapeutic nature (when there is a risk to the mother, and in the detection of malformations and other anomalies). This country has the highest percentage of doctors, obstetricians or anesthesiologists, around 70%, who refuse to perform this procedure. (**)

Since 1977, abortion in New Zealand has been allowed up to twenty weeks of pregnancy, and after twenty weeks if it harms the woman's health. The regulations require that abortions after twelve weeks of pregnancy must be carried out in hospitals (**)

In Australia, abortion has been legalized since 1970. The progressive increase in the number of women being exposed to this procedure has prompted the Australian government to initiate an education program to prevent this increase in abortions.

In Mogambique, abortion was regulated by law, and was only allowed if the pregnant woman's life was at risk. With the new Penal Code, abortion was allowed up to twelve weeks of pregnancy, and in the case of rape, up to the sixteenth week. This law was promulgated by Mogambican President Armando Guebuza in December 2014. (**)

During Mandela's rule in the Republic of South Africa, abortion was made free. There are private clinics, but the government offers it free of charge. Up to the twelfth week, the procedure is medicated. (**)

On the African continent, in addition to the Republic of South Africa and Mogambique, Cape Verde and Tunisia are other countries where abortion legislation exists. (**)

By citing events in different countries with different religious majorities, varying geographical locations and opposing political organizations, we can understand that the liberation or restriction of abortion takes place in a more social and political field than a scientific one. This is because, in terms of surgical risk for the pregnant woman, the risk is very small.

Rodrigues Torres, a law judge, in an article comparing the laws of various nations in the 21st century, gives an overview of the situation in the European Union: (25)

a) prohibition of abortion without exception: Malta;
b) abortion allowed at the woman's request, with a certain gestation period (from 90 days to 24 weeks); United Kingdom, Netherlands, Sweden, Romania, Denmark, Latvia, Czech Republic, Slovakia, Greece, Hungary, Belgium, Bulgaria, France, Germany, Lithuania, Estonia, Portugal, Slovenia, Austria and Italy;
c) abortion is always permitted if the pregnant woman's life is at risk: United Kingdom, Denmark, Sweden, Latvia, Poland, Slovenia, Austria, Czech Republic, Slovakia, Romania, Cyprus, Greece, Hungary, Spain, Portugal, France, Germany, Lithuania, Estonia, Luxembourg and Ireland (includes risk of suicide);
d) abortion allowed if the pregnant woman's life is at risk, with a certain gestation period: the Netherlands and Finland;
e) abortion is always permitted if there is a risk to the health of the pregnant woman: Denmark, Slovenia, Austria, Czech Republic, Slovakia, Romania, Cyprus, Hungary, Belgium, Italy, France and Germany;
(f) abortion permitted on the grounds of risk to the health of the pregnant woman, with a certain length of gestation (from 90 days to 28 weeks): Lithuania, Latvia, the Netherlands, the United Kingdom, Estonia, Ireland, Luxembourg, Portugal, Poland and Spain;

g) abortion is allowed when the pregnancy is the result of rape or another sexual crime, always: Romania, Cyprus, Greece, Germany and Hungary;
h) abortion is allowed when the pregnancy is the result of rape or another sexual crime with a certain gestation period (from 90 days to 28 weeks): Denmark, Finland, France, Spain, Belgium, Poland, Italy, Luxembourg, Portugal, Lithuania, Estonia, the Netherlands, and Latvia;
i) abortion allowed when there is fetal malformation, with no gestation period requirement: United Kingdom, Austria, Czech Republic, Slovakia, Romania, Cyprus, Hungary, France, Germany and Bulgaria;
j) abortion allowed when there is a fetal malformation, with a certain gestation period: Holland, Denmark, Sweden, Finland, Latvia, Estonia and Luxembourg;
k) "abortion allowed for socio-economic reasons with a certain gestation period: the Netherlands, Finland, Italy, France and Luxembourg." (25)

This work also contains a passage on the nations of Latin America:

Cuba, which in 1965 legalized abortion up to 12 weeks gestation, maintains a lower abortion rate of 21 per thousand women of reproductive age, ten points below the regional average.
Chile, El Salvador, Nicaragua and the Dominican Republic have criminalized abortion and do not allow exceptions.
Honduras, because of the Code of Medical Ethics, allows abortion to save the life of the pregnant woman.
Argentina, Costa Rica, Venezuela, Peru and Paraguay allow abortion to save the woman's life. and in Venezuela to protect the honor of the woman and the man.
Uruguay, Colombia, Ecuador, Bolivia, Mexico, Panama and Guatemala allow abortion in cases of rape or incest. Uruguay also allows it in cases of economic distress and Colombia, Mexico and Panama allow it in cases of fetal malformation (25).

Brazil maintains the criminalization of non-punishable abortion in cases of rape or when there is no other way to save the life of the pregnant woman.

However, the internationally validated human rights system has already recognized that women have the right to freely determine the number of their children and the intervals between their births, and to decide over their own bodies.

This shows how variable the different nations' approach is to the treatment of abortion. Different cultures take the same approach, while others differ sharply.

Societies have different concerns about abortion, as do the different strata. This can be demonstrated by the work that has been done and will now be shared.

A respectable part of the medical elite of the state of Sao Paulo is to be found in the Sao Paulo Academy of Medicine. (16) This is the state with the largest population, the highest economic productivity, the best university institutions in South America, and health and disease care is provided in the most advanced institutions in the country and placed on an equal level with the best in the world. When academics were asked what legislation on abortion should be considered and established in Brazil, a survey carried out in mid-2015 revealed some aspects (16).

Eight conditions were asked in order to choose the desired one. They were as follows:

1. I agree with the current legislation in Brazil, which does not punish the crime of abortion if the woman is raped, if her life is in danger or if the fetus is anencephalic.

2. I agree with the proposal put forward by the Federal Council of Medicine not to punish abortions in pregnant women up to the 12th week of pregnancy.

3 I agree with the WHO statement that abortion should be made easier for pregnant women infected with the Zika virus.

4 I agree that abortion should be completely free if it is the woman's wish to undergo it and the doctor's wish to perform it.

5. I have no opinion on the matter.

6. I am against abortion at any time.

7. I don't want to reveal my opinion.

8. Other.

In a universe of 123 academics, 109 male and 14 female, 47 responses were received, which corresponded to 38.2% of the total number of members, 44 from male members, i.e. 40.3%, and 3 from female members, which shows a percentage of 21.4. Even in a subject that is essentially female, women responded in a much lower percentage than the percentage of responses received from men. In reality, when there is no reciprocation for an answer, the lack of responses is high.

The first insight gained from this survey is the low level of concern about the issue shown by members of an important
institution, which brings together the cream of the world's most advanced medicine.
The percentage of responses to the various questions was:
1 I agree with the current legislation in Brazil, which does not punish the crime of abortion if the woman is raped, if there is no other way to save the woman's life or if the fetus is anencephalic. 11 (eleven)

2. I agree with the proposal put forward by the Federal Council of Medicine that abortion in pregnant women up to the 12th week of pregnancy should not be punished. 3 (three)

3 I agree with the WHO statement that abortion should be made easier for pregnant women infected with the Zika virus. 7(seven)

4 I agree that abortion should be completely free if it is the woman's wish to undergo it and the doctor's wish to perform it. 10 (ten).

5. I have no opinion on the matter. (0) zero.

6. I am against abortion at any time. 5 (five).

7. I do not wish to reveal my opinion. (0) zero.

8. Other. 0 (zero).

Eleven answers were divided between more than one question. These were the questions and the respective indications of the answers.

1 and 2: 1 (one); 1 and 3: 4 (four); 1 and 8: 1 (one);
1, 2 and 3: 1 (one); 2, 3 and 4: 3 (three); 2 and 3: 1 (one).

Looking at the answers, it is not possible to make any statements defining the academics' positions. What is worth noting is that 11 (eleven) academics who offered to reveal their positions said that they did not have a firm position, agreeing with more than one of the questions.

Another 11 (eleven) agreed with the current legislation of the Brazilian Penal Code which considers abortion a crime, only not punishable under special conditions: rape or if there is no other way to save the woman's life. Another 7 (seven) included item 1 along with others, making a total of 18 (eighteen).

Ten (10) considered that abortion can be performed if the woman wishes to undergo it and the doctor agrees to perform it. Another 3 (three) included this item along with others, totaling

13 (thirteen).

The appeal by the World Health Organization suggesting a reduction in restrictions on abortion when the woman is proven to be infected with the Zika virus was the position mentioned by 7 (seven). Another 9 (nine) included this item together with another, for a total of 16 (sixteen).

The opinion of the Federal Code of Medicine that abortion should be performed up to the 12th week was the answer given by 3 (three) academics. Another 6 (six) included this item along with others, making a total of 9 (nine).

Five (5) academics agreed against abortion in any situation.

After analyzing these responses, it is not possible to mention any position of the members of the Sao Paulo Academy of Medicine, because a majority of members refused to answer the survey, even though they were warned that their responses would be considered anonymous. In fact, in another survey of opinion on another social medical aspect, that is, the possibility of practicing orthotanasia, with the universe of members of the Sao Paulo Academy of Medicine, in 2010, 39 (thirty-nine) out of 92 (ninety-two) respondents answered, which corresponded to 42.4%.

Among those who responded, there was no trend indicating a position, but rather different positions.

"In a debatable subject, which for health involves legal, ethical and religious aspects, as well as bioethical ones, involving discussions of autonomy and heteronomy, when a biological being is a person, the beginning of life, the inviolability of life and other aspects, we haven't found a marked concern among doctors of a higher caliber. It is possible.

to admit that the social aspects of health care in general are not of interest to doctors, but rather matters exclusive to their specialties. On the other hand, it must be considered that in the culture of the Brazilian people, the problem of abortion is not a major concern." (16).

This ambiguous position is found in the culture of Brazilian society, which in general does not agree with abortion, nor does it punish those who perform it. (16)
Other studies give the same interpretation.

A study carried out in the city of Santos, State of Sao Paulo, Brazil, in 1973, with a probabilistic sample of fertile, married women portrays aspects of fertility and contraception. (13)
Santos is a coastal city located approximately 80 kilometers west of the city of Sao Paulo, the capital of the state of Sao Paulo, and linked to it by road and rail. At the time it had a population of around 350,000 inhabitants with a population density of 720 inhabitants per square kilometer. The largest export port in South America was in the city. Although it was the largest seaside town in the state, it was also the center of an important industrial zone with an oil refinery, hydroelectric power station, shipyards and port warehouses. The population is made up of different ethnic groups, typical of the state of São Paulo, but with a strong emphasis on Portuguese ancestry, as well as the presence of Italian and Spanish descendants.
A carefully surveyed sample began with a detailed, up-to-date map of the city and using a table of randomized numbers, 50 blocks were chosen at random. In each block, 10 households were chosen, using a previously established procedure, that had a woman with a marital life, aged up to 49. This sample represented 0.7 percent of the women living in Santos.
Of the 500 households selected and visited, it was possible to collect data from 470. The positive response rate was 94%. There was no geographical or urban difference between the households in which the women did or did not answer the interviewers.
As far as abortion is concerned, the answers obtained showed data referring to spontaneous abortions and induced abortions. 24.3% of the women interviewed reported having had a spontaneous abortion. 15.5% reported having caused at least one abortion. Of all the women interviewed, 32.6% reported having had an abortion.

A more modern study updating the estimates of induced abortion in Brazil between 1995 and 2013 provides important data. (18)
Using the number of hospitalizations as the primary data source
by abortion registered in the Hospital Information System of the Brazilian Unified Health System. Using this methodology, this study considered the percentage of 12.5% for under-registration cases and the proportion of 25% for spontaneous abortions.

In 2010, a National Abortion Survey was carried out: "Abortion in Brazil: a household survey with ballot box technique" (7).
The article summarizes "the first results of the National Abortion Survey, a random sample survey of households carried out in 2010, covering women aged

between 18 and 39 throughout urban Brazil. This survey combined two polling techniques: the ballot box technique and questionnaires completed by female interviewers. The results indicate that, by the end of their reproductive lives, more than one in five women have had an abortion, with abortions generally occurring at the ages that make up the center of women's reproductive period, i.e. between 18 and 29. There was no significant difference in practice according to religious belief, but abortion was more common among women with less schooling."

These results lead the authors to conclude that abortion should be a priority on the national public health agenda. The authors state that "the National Abortion Survey combined two polling techniques, the ballot box technique and questionnaires completed by interviewers, to collect data on abortion in urban Brazil from a stratified sample of 2,002 literate women aged between 18 and 39 in 2010. The results refer to women who have had abortions, not abortions. The number of abortions in the country is higher than that counted by the survey, not only because the same woman can have more than one abortion, but also because illiterate women and rural areas of Brazil were not covered by the survey. The PNA indicates that abortion is so common in Brazil that, by the age of forty, more than one in five women have had an abortion. Typically, abortions take place in the middle of the female reproductive period, i.e. between the ages of 18 and 29, and are more common among women with lower levels of education, a fact that may be related to other social characteristics of women with low levels of education.

Religion is not an important factor in differentiating women when it comes to having abortions. Reflecting the religious composition of the country, the majority of abortions were performed by Catholics, followed by Protestants and Evangelicals, and finally by women of other religions or no religion. The use of medication to induce the last abortion occurred in half of the cases. Considering that most of the women have a low level of education, it is likely that for the other half of the women, who did not use medication, the abortion was carried out under poor health conditions. Not surprisingly, the levels of post-abortion hospitalization recorded by the study are high, occurring in almost half of the cases." The authors conclude that such a common phenomenon with such important health consequences places abortion high on the national public health agenda (7).

As a result, this study shows that 22% of older women aged 35 to 39 have had an abortion. (7)

In another study carried out with medical and law students enrolled at the University of Sao Paulo, Brazil, it is impossible to say whether the culture of the city's society accepts or rejects the practice of abortion. (14) The students chosen were chosen for the following reasons:
1. Students from areas linked to health and legislation, i.e. students who would, by the nature of their professional field, have to deal with the issue of abortion, either in the medical or legal spheres.
2. Students who are in their fourth year could already have a more professional opinion, even if incipient, about the problem of abortion; in addition, they would also be close to entering the job market, which means that the results obtained in the

survey were indicators of the tendency of opinion of those who would soon be professionals working in areas related to abortion;
3. Young students who, in a way, could be personally involved, more or less intensely, with the issue of abortion.

Among the medical students, 92 were male and 59 female; 148 were single and the average age was 21.7 years. 4 did not state their gender.
Among the law students, 72 were male and 68 female; 133 were single and the average age was 21.8 years. One student did not state his gender.
The opinion survey was carried out using a questionnaire handed out in class without any suggestions for answers. Statistically analyzed at 5%, the responses obtained from medical and law students showed no differences, nor were any significant differences found between the genres.
The overall result showed that 6 students (2.1%) had no answers, 142 (48.4%) were in favor of liberation and 148 (49.5%) were against it.

With the creation of the Unified Health System in Brazil and the attention being paid to women who claimed to have been raped, even though the rapists had not yet been convicted by the courts, some other information could be obtained. The Unified Health System has set up a service in a public hospital for these pregnant women, offering the possibility of terminating unwanted pregnancies.
The fact that these surveys were carried out, collecting data on abortion, demonstrates the idea that for Brazilian society the fact of having had an abortion does not characterize a woman in any way.

What we learn as we go through history is that abortion, liberated or penalized according to culture, is always found as a social practice.
Legislation in all countries has changed more rapidly, some more slowly, in line with the changes that have taken place in cultures as a result of scientific and social changes.

4 Man on earth

In order to make an analysis that allows for reflection, it is necessary to set out a few aspects. It should be remembered that for centuries, ever since man has been known to live on earth, life has been considered to have originated from the divine breath of gods. Gods, of different rituals, from the mystical ones, characteristic of the staple peoples, to those of greater pomp found in so many churches. These various rituals include the giving of offerings, ranging from prayers to lives. Gods, however, have always served to explain, in a complete and dogmatic way, what happens to the supernatural, exactly what human knowledge does not know and is not in a position to make categorical statements about.

As much as scientific knowledge brings news about when man has his current constitution, what his beginnings are, what his possible evolution from other animals is, the questions to these issues present answers that are always controversial. Those who think rationally, based on scientific values, have positions on man and his presence that emerged in confrontations from the mid-nineteenth century onwards. These recent ideas, compared to the times of humanity, have the force of modernity and the conviction of the most literate. It is reason that stands before faith. Scientists of all stripes are arguing with believers from all churches.

In the Holy Bible, in the Old Testament, in what is the first book of the Pentateuch, (1) the book of origins, Genesis, we read: "In the beginning God created the heaven and the earth" and further on in the same book we find: "And God said, Let us make man in our image and after our likeness; and he shall rule over the fish of the sea, and over the fowl of the air, and over the beasts, and over all creeping things that move upon the earth, and have dominion over all the earth. And God created man in his own image: he made him in the image of God, and created them male and female". According to the theory of evolution (**) proposed by Darwin, now considered by many to be completely verified in all its purposes and meanings, and by Marcel Blanc to have given rise to many controversies, living beings are related to each other and have had a common ancestor at some point since the emergence of life. The origin of life occurred more than a billion years ago.

Despite the depth of the studies and the information obtained to date, there is still no unequivocal evidence to suggest that these theories, which translate the presence of man in the various moments of his life on earth, are irrefutable.

The theory of evolution was accepted by the elites, the scholars and the scientists, while the lower classes continued to believe in the different gods encouraged by priests who, regardless of their beliefs, always had one or more gods to worship.

There is no fully accepted theory explaining how man appeared on earth. There are various religious doctrines followed by those who believe in them, or in other words, what the belief makes you accept and thus satisfies you as an explanation for something that hasn't been explained, let alone demonstrated or proven. These are the sacred mysteries of beliefs and believers.

For those who don't believe, Darwin came along at the end of the 19th century with his theory of evolution. (**) Darwin showed that the human lineage was the result of evolutionary pressures at work for millions of years, just as much as any other living being. Darwin's ideas, however, fell by the wayside, perhaps because they were understandable only to the elites. In his theory, he proposed that all living beings, from the wisest of men to the single-celled bacillus, could have their ancestral lineage traced back to the beginning of life on Earth. This proposal, however, was not in line with religious preaching, which called for divine reasons.

Before Darwin, science was twisted around the religious belief that all living things had been created by God and that it was up to man to give them names. Before Darwin, no scientist had the arguments and intellectual courage to oppose the religious idea of creation. Discoveries and inventions were pathetically adapted to religious dogma. That's why it seems plausible that at one point in history, conservative Catholic culture opposed Darwin's theory, while Protestant and liberal culture accepted it.

When the bones of dinosaurs and other extinct animals began to be unearthed, the French savant Georges Cuvier offered the most extraordinary of these adaptations: "They are the bones of animals that were unable to board Noah's Ark and died in the biblical flood." (**)

Darwin broke this paradigm and clashed head-on with the Protestant and Catholic religious hierarchy. He did so in a calm but irrefutable manner. Darwin's theory is that the living world was neither created nor perpetually recycled and that organisms are in a slow but constant   process of change   .
that every group of organisms descends from a common ancestor. Today's humans and apes, for example, diverged from the same ancestor around 4 million years ago.

All living things are ultimately descended from a simple, primitive form of life - the so-called "original amoeba". (**)

Darwin, however, was unable to explain where this so-called "original amoeba" originated. If there is an evolution in the creation of living beings, who created the first of them?

Living species tend to differentiate with the passage of time. Darwin drew the first "tree of life" in which "trunk" species give rise to others that emerge from the main vein as "branches" (**)

Again the same question: Darwin drew the tree of life. Who gave rise to that tree?

Doubts that neither Darwin nor the scientists who followed his theory were able to provide complete answers to.

In Darwin's theory, populations gradually differentiate, from generation to generation, until the species that have followed one "branch" of the tree of life no longer belong to the same species as the "trunk" and other "branches". (**) It is based on the fact that living beings undergo genetic mutations and can pass them on to their descendants. Each new generation has its genetic inheritance put to the test by the environmental conditions in which it lives. Evolution is opportunistic and random. Mutations occur at random, and not with the aim of improving the survival chances of those who suffer them. A simple example: primitive fish could not draw oxygen directly from the water. Some underwent mutations that endowed them with this ability. The latter adapted better to aquatic life and today dominate rivers, lakes and oceans. (**)

It's a scientific theory. As such, it can be dismantled as long as a single piece of evidence emerges that it doesn't work. Darwin said that if someone pointed out to him a single living being that didn't have an ancestor, his theory could be thrown in the garbage can. The neo-Darwinists are even more defiant: if you can prove that a single organ of a living being (eyes, ears, fins...) did not originate from a proto-organ (eyes, ears, primitive fins), the whole Darwinian theory can be thrown out. (**)

If Darwin hadn't proposed the theory of evolution, he would still be remembered as one of humanity's geniuses. His works on experimental botany, animal psychology and classification are still required reading for scholars today. Many pre-Darwinists paved the way for Darwin, especially with regard to gradualism. The ancient Greeks and Chinese accepted that life forms could change over time or even disappear.

Alfred Russel Wallace, a contemporary of Darwin, independently developed a theory of evolution. (**) What made Darwin unique was the rigor of his scientific method, his multidisciplinary capacity,
in addition to the disciplined process of obtaining and drawing conclusions. (**)

After the original impact of his ideas, Darwin wrote that both present-day humans and apes had primitive ancestors. But this has been the most resistant falsehood about Darwinism. Darwin undoubtedly showed that the human lineage is the result of evolutionary pressures at work for millions of years, just as much as any other living being. In later editions of his work *The Origin of Species...,* Darwin suggested that living beings could pass on acquired characteristics to their descendants. Darwin faced fierce opposition from traditional scientific institutions, as well as disbelief and terrible family pressures. In this environment, it is not strange that Darwin flirted with processes that were less offensive to religious dogma. In fact, Darwin's wife feared that when both she and Darwin died, she would go to heaven and he to hell.

Darwin is recognized for his ideas, but his theory of human evolution, although valuable for its originality, has not yet reached a majority of scientists that would make it absolutely valid. Originating at the end of the nineteenth century, the theory of evolution lasted throughout the twentieth century, practically without any major modifications and without provoking any major enthusiasm in scientific circles. It's worth remembering that in the twentieth century, man on earth saw the appearance of electricity, which brought about phenomenal illumination, and from earth, man went to the moon and reached Mars with rockets in the twenty-first century.

Nowadays, no one is frightened by the possibility that the theory of the Origin of Species is correct, but it is the reason for many disagreements and discussions.

The future can bring everything, but man's origin lies more in the proclamations of religious divinities than in the discoveries of science.

5 The beginning of life

The approach that different nations take to the treatment of abortion varies. Different cultures take the same approach, while others differ sharply.

These changes between nations have their origins in when life is considered to begin. The first contradiction is when a biological being, the product of a couple's fertilization, should be considered a person, fulfilling the physical, psychological and social conditions that characterize it as such. When it comes to the development of techniques based on knowledge from the health sciences, there is a natural involvement with aspects of people's lives. In the discussion about life, especially when it comes to its beginning or its preservation, reason is confronted with emotion and faith. Bioethical reflections have a role to play precisely in this confrontation, seeking to establish what course should be taken while respecting the modernism of the avant-garde, but not forgetting the conservatism of traditional values. (15)

The opposing positions, represented on the one hand by those who defend the principle of autonomy and on the other by those who argue in favor of heteronomy, prevent the possibility of a dialogue capable of leading, if not to consensus, to a conciliatory situation.

The beginning of life is a concern that is always being discussed, especially from a religious perspective. Life is a continuum that has never ceased to exist since its inception. (15) What is debated is when a complex caused by a union of biological cells becomes or is considered a person. This is a question that dates back to the mythological times of Asclepius, Aristotle and Hippocrates and which has not been definitively resolved to this day.

According to various cultures in different societies, in which religious values, doctrines and dogmas of the various existing religions predominate, the beginning of life occurs at the moment of conception, i.e. at the union of the male spermatozoon with the female ovum. Other more liberal beliefs consider different and diverse occasions.

For many (12), the biological being that comes from the union of the male and female gametes of human beings is considered a person when it has fulfilled three conditions:

1. In the ecological field: in relation to the environment in which you will live;
2. In the social field: in relation to the people you'll be living with;
3. 3. In the spiritual realm: in relation to the natural realm, whether in the institutionalized form of religious churches or any other form, but guided by a form of values in which you will believe.

In times gone by, the idea that a new life began when the ovum was fertilized, if it was disseminated in scientific and ethical circles, and if it wasn't, it wasn't fully accepted. It was the word of the religious that predominated.

Concern about the issue gained momentum when, in 1798, Malthus raised the link between population and the economy. Some countries took the issue to the 5th World Health Assembly, provoking discussions. In response to the concern about population growth, which was considered undesirable, certain nations began to encourage birth control using the methods known at the time, which began with having sex only during safe periods, using the Ogino Knauss table or using a mechanical condom known as Condon. (15)

The use of intrauterine devices, known from more distant times, employed by the Arabs who placed stones in the uterus of she-camels when they set out on long desert treks, only began to be used more widely from 1928. The acceptance of intrauterine methods from 1960 onwards raised the protest of religious and theologians who considered them abortifacients. However, studies have shown that around 50% of fertilized eggs are found in women's normal menstruation. This knowledge led to the hypothesis that fertilization required more than the union of an egg and sperm. It would take not only fertilization, but also the attachment of the egg to the endometrium of the uterus. With the knowledge brought about by these studies, it was considered that the emergence of another human being could only occur not at fertilization, but at nesting. As a result, society's ethical position has changed, with the exception of the religious, who persist in considering the emergence of human life from conception.

With the birth in 1978 of the first artificially fertilized child, after a long controversy between those in favor and those opposed to this methodology, new positions were taken on the subject of the beginning of life. (15)

The development of this methodology today allows the birth of a child by the method of artificial fertilization, with the gamete of a man, not necessarily the husband or partner of the woman who offers the female gamete, which after being artificially fertilized will be placed in the uterus of a second woman or in the woman herself, in which the pregnancy will proceed. Recently, a technique that is only allowed to be used in the UK has been carried out in Mexico by American scientists: mitochondrial transfer, which allows fertilization with the presence of a third person, i.e. using mitochondria from a healthy woman. This advance is not yet common knowledge. Thus, science develops new techniques and methods to meet health needs, which are not always accompanied by ethical codes or the relevant legislation.

In Brazil, since 1984, when the first child fertilized by this technology was born, the use of the artificial fertilization method has been successful, as in many other countries in the world, which makes it impossible to recognize the children born this way. (15)

However, it wasn't until the International Conference on Population and Development in Cairo in 1994 that the issue of abortion came to the fore. This conference is considered a milestone on abortion. In Cairo, for the first time, an inter-ministerial forum recognized that abortion complications pose serious threats to public health and recommended that, where access to abortion is not against the law, it should be carried out under safe conditions. (**)

On many occasions during artificial fertilization techniques, a larger number of embryos develop during embryo transfers. The technique advocates the reduction of embryos that will be discarded or frozen for a maximum period of five years and then disposed of. The question arises as to whether this technique can be considered abortive, at least for those who consider the embryo to be a human being from the moment of fertilization.

Still on the subject of when life begins, there is a need to consider when life begins.
Another theory should be borne in mind, which argues that a person's personality begins at birth. This is the case in Eastern nations, where attention to the new being only becomes concrete with birth.

6 Sacred life

This discussion is fundamental, because it is the basis for opinions on whether or not to consecrate life. It is a polemic: whether the greater importance lies in the consecration or in the quality of life. This brings together what Engelhardt (8) says when he says that "the moral life is lived in two dimensions." It is not intended to enter into a debate about whether secular ethics or canonical ethics should prevail. Religious positions are accepted and accepted, but alongside religious positions, especially those of the Catholic Church, some incongruities are revealed, such as those who are against the possibility of allowing abortion, but accept the use of assisted reproduction techniques in which embryos are discarded. It's worth remembering that in the seventies of the last century, the idea of assisted fertilization was reprehensible, as it is now, and the liberation of abortion is still restricted.

When it comes to abortion, there are ethical positions.

One is that of those who deny the possibility of abortion under any condition, which is the position defended by preachers of the Catholic religion, and others (9) who consider that a person's life begins at conception, i.e. when the sperm meets the ovum. This is very close to the position of devotees of other churches who believe that a person's life begins at different times, but before birth, as preached by groups of followers of Judaism and Islam. Others, however, consider that a person's life begins at birth, i.e. when the biological being has a social position in society as a person. (15) These positions are products of the faith that human beings have in the dogmas of their religion. It is not for us to discuss them, but rather to respect them. However, it should be noted that Gafo, a Spanish Catholic priest, states in one of his writings that the Bible does not clearly or explicitly condemn abortion. (15)

Another position is the acceptance of abortion, either with restrictions or with freedom. This is undoubtedly currently the majority position worldwide. If abortion is carried out with an acceptable justification, society does not sanction it in any way. Variations occur in the type of justification, ranging up to strict requirements that almost prevent it from being carried out, as is the case with Brazilian legislation (3). Among the justifications, the ones with the strongest repercussions are the so-called therapeutic abortions, i.e. abortions carried out to save the life of the pregnant woman, and eugenic abortions carried out when the fetus has anomalies.

These justifications are supported by the defense of women's health. Justifications for social reasons are not mentioned, but for social reasons, countless women seek abortion and carry it out illegally.

In Brazil, abortion is a crime for which the doctor and the pregnant woman under special conditions provided for in the Penal Code are not punished.

The law does not provide for what is known here as sentimental rape and it is not always discussed. This is when a man, without using physical violence or serious threats, manages, through promises and oaths of love, to maintain a sexual relationship with a woman who, once the pregnancy is proven, abandons him. This is different from fraud, because on many occasions, before the woman became pregnant, the man had no intention of abandoning his partner, nor did he act without the woman's consent. He abandons her because he doesn't want to take on paternity, unlike fraud when the intention to abandon is the man's goal from the outset, even before the woman's pregnancy or without the worry of pregnancy.

Discussing the fact of permission for the act, which, however, is similar to the fact that it is not punishable when the woman is incapable of understanding the relationship. She does not understand the fact when she is intellectually incapable, or when she is under 14. She does not understand when she is deceived.

The birth of anencephalic babies has led to discussion about the possibility of terminating pregnancies in such cases. (5)
In April 2012, the Supreme Court ruled that aborting a fetus without a brain is not a crime.

The emergence of cases of Zika, a disease caused by a virus from the Flavavirus family, which was found in 1947 in Uganda, Africa, and has now spread to South America and Africa, has caused concern among public health officials in these regions. Transmission between people is mainly through the Aedes aegypti mosquito. Sexual transmission is also considered a route for this disease. Because the first cases of this virus were observed in monkeys in a place called Zika, the factor and the disease were given this name. Zika is a relatively mild disease with mild symptoms that can include joint, muscle and head pain and a not very high fever. Its treatment is aimed at reducing the symptoms. Since 2015, the presence of this disease in South America has increased, with a greater prevalence in Brazil. A serious consequence of this disease is the possibility of a pregnant woman being affected by the virus and the product of the fetus being born with microcephaly and a reduced skull.

The World Health Organization has been very concerned about this. People living in areas where local transmission of the Zika virus occurs should therefore also practice safe sex or abstain from sexual activity. On the other hand, people returning from areas where local transmission of Zika virus occurs should adopt safer sex practices or abstain from sexual intercourse for at least eight weeks after their return, even if they have no symptoms. If men have symptoms of Zika virus, they should adopt safer sex practices or consider abstinence for at least six months. Women planning a pregnancy should wait at least eight weeks before trying to conceive if there are no symptoms of Zika virus infection, or six months if one or both members of the couple have symptoms.

Despite these warnings and the concern not to get pregnant unwillingly and in the face of Brazilian legislation, Rodrigo Janot, Attorney General of the Brazilian Republic, made a statement defending the release of abortion in cases of pregnant women carrying the Zika virus. The issue has once again prompted Brazilian society to speak out on the matter. (19)

In a statement addressed to the Supreme Court, the President of the Federal Senate Renan Calheiros, through the Senate Advocate's Office, claims that abortion in these circumstances is a matter of sharp ethical dissent on which parliamentarians are unlikely to adopt uniform positions. The argument was presented in the context of the lawsuit filed by the National Association of Public Defenders asking for the right to abortion for women infected with the Zika virus. The Brazilian Senate was summoned by Justice Carmen Lucia, the rapporteur of the case, to make a statement. The

Attorney General's Office, which defends the interests of the federal government, argues that terminating the pregnancy would violate the right to life. (19)

Today's knowledge of fetal medicine allows a fetus to be operated on, just as it allows a fetus to be diagnosed with anencephaly or microcephaly. The evolution of scientific knowledge is clearly not accompanied by changes in legislation, and for this to happen we need courageous decisions that generate debate.

Microcephaly is to be examined by the Supreme Court, according to a statement by Carmem Lucia, President of the Brazilian Supreme Court.

Demonstrating a trend on the matter, the 1st Panel of the Superior Federal Court, on November 29, 2016, in a decision that took into account women's reproductive rights, ruled for a case involving employees and doctors of a clandestine clinic in Duque de Caxias, RJ. that voluntary termination of pregnancy carried out in the first trimester of pregnancy is not a crime.

The judicial decision known to the Chamber of Deputies led to the interruption of discussions on other matters in order to hear some protests, which provoked the President of the collegiate body to set up a specific Committee to study and pronounce on the matter.

Dom Odilo P. Scherer (2) said: "*It is not a question of freeing abortion in general, nor of its pure and simple decriminalization. However, the decision creates a precedent that can be invoked and applied by judges in other similar cases. It has opened the way for "legal" abortions to be carried out before three months of pregnancy have elapsed. *"

For this discussion, it is necessary to bring to light the thoughts of those who, even though they are attached to religious postulates, understand that these positions must change.

Odilo P. Scherer is a Brazilian cardinal, the nineteenth bishop of Sao Paulo, Brazil, his seventh archbishop and fifth cardinal. The son of Edwino Scherer and Francisca Wilma Steffens Scherer, he is a descendant of German immigrants from the *Saarland* region who settled in Rio Grande do Sul. He is the sixth child of the couple, out of a total of 13 siblings. He is a distant relative of the late Cardinal Dom Vicente Scherer.

Concerned about social life in general, in addition to his Catholic devotion, Dom Odilo published an article in April 2013 in the newspaper O Estado de S.Paulo (22) in which he analyzed the reasons for abortion, putting forward the position of the Catholic Church.

He began by saying that in view of the decision of the Federal Council of Medicine in favor of abortion up to the 12th week of pregnancy, depending only on the woman's autonomous will, an opportunity was offered to address the issue. The opportunity to deal with the issue was favorable, but the favorable decision of the Federal Council of Medicine is debatable, as no resolution to this effect has been published.

It presents reasons to affirm that in human life it is not possible to have a phase that is not human from fertilization when the sperm unites with the ovum, a moment that the Catholic Church recognizes as the beginning of the life of a human being.

Therefore, in the 13th week of pregnancy, according to Dom Odilio, a living human being already exists from fertilization onwards. There is no reason to allow abortion up to the 12th week of pregnancy, even in a secular state, because human rights exist for everyone, regardless of their beliefs.

In his article, Dom Odilo discusses the abortion situation in countries that are considered more developed, where the possibility for women to undergo abortion much more liberally is evident. (22)

The article ends by stating that this is not a religious situation, but a human rights one, and that there would only be one way to change this view if the unborn fetus were not considered human.

Those who believe that life is sacred consider the inviolability of life and do not refer to the quality of life are against abortion. Performing an abortion constitutes murder of an unborn child. (10)

7 The quality of life

On all occasions other than those established by legislation, abortion in Brazil is carried out in the shadows. Social groups, including doctors, claim a wide range of justifications for abortion, especially when there are fetuses with abnormalities, which would lead them to suffer and not last long after birth. This last point is a good example of the difference between those who consider life to be sacred and those who think it's more important to know about the quality of life. What quality of life can a woman recognized as poor have to raise a child if she is abandoned by the child's father? Why can a woman, regardless of her socio-economic situation, have an abortion for legal or biological reasons? This is the fundamental dilemma in this matter. Although in the minority, those who defend a position against the liberation of abortion have the strength of the churches and divine dogma.

In the Encyclical "The Gospel of Life" Pope John Paul II does not fail to understand that some women who find it very difficult to avoid abortion are not automatically sent to hell. The Encyclical reads:

"It's true that the choice to abort often has a dramatic and painful character for the mother: the decision to dispose of the conceived child is not taken for purely selfish reasons or for convenience, but because they want to safeguard important goods such as their own health or a decent standard of living for the other members of the family. Sometimes, the unborn child's fear of the living conditions he or she will have to face leads him or her to think that it would be better not to be born. But these and similar reasons, however serious and dramatic, can never justify the deliberate elimination of an innocent human being. When deciding on the death of an unborn child, not only the mother but also the father of the child appear as guilty parties, not only when he forces the woman to have an abortion or indirectly favors such a decision by leaving her alone "

The Pope describes, without justifying the decision, why a woman often prefers abortion to having a child who will not be able to offer her at least a reasonable quality of life. Other situations must also be considered: when the father is unknown; when the family can throw her out of the house; when there are no conditions to support the child; when the fetus is abnormal.

Just as the violence of rape, the absence of means to save the woman's life, and the presence of an abnormal fetus are used to justify not considering an abortion a crime, we should understand the social reasons for the same justification.

Modern artificial fertilization procedures already select healthy embryos to be fertilized, and the rest are discarded. Isn't it incongruous to accept this procedure and take a stand against abortion?

These facts mean that data on abortions is unknown due to the illegality of practicing them. However, through surveys of pregnancy histories, it is possible to estimate that approximately a quarter of fertile, sexually active women suffer an abortion in their lifetime. Half of these abortions are almost always caused by precarious conditions. Precariousness in the health conditions in which the surgical procedure is carried out and precariousness in the psychological accompaniment of the woman who proposes to undergo it.

Four women die every day in Brazil from abortion complications, and this statistic would be greatly reduced if there were no criminal restrictions on abortion.

The Federal Council of Medicine (6), commenting on the reform of the Brazilian Penal Code, recommends that abortion in women up to twelve weeks pregnant should not be punished as a crime, as has been the case in countless other countries for more than half a century.

It must be understood that the quality of life does not result exclusively from the lawfulness of the birth or from abortion being carried out under ethical or religious precepts. The quality of life concerns the social formation of the family alongside the possible biological quality of the child to be born. In the absence of any of these social or physical conditions, the quality of life is diminished. It is up to the woman who becomes pregnant to decide. It seems that only she will be able to judge, in the light of these variables, whether it is worth bringing the fetus to life. The single mother or the child who doesn't have a father doesn't have a full quality of life in the eyes of society, which, on the other hand, has nothing to do with a woman who has had an abortion.

8 Religions and abortion

There are contradictions among the followers of the religions that spread throughout society. It is estimated that there are more than three thousand sects and doctrines that have their dogmas, their particularities and their essences, from which they do not differ.

In reality, the predominant religion in the Western world, and especially in Latin countries, is Catholicism, alongside the various doctrines that are attached to Christianity.

In the Western world, the Jewish religion is also widespread, with its center in Jerusalem in the State of Israel.

Eastern countries are followers of other religions such as Buddhism, Islam and Hinduism.

Buddhism and its offshoots are mostly located in Japan.

Islam is predominant in Iraq and the Arab countries.

Hinduism is practically located in India, Nepal, Pakistan and Sri Lanka.

Catholicism, as a religion, dominated the Western world for the first fifteen hundred years after Christ's presence on earth. In 1517, Martin Luther, a friar of the Order of St. Augustine, promoted a great movement to break the unity of the Church. The Reformation also touched on political and social aspects, causing conflicts in Europe. In a broader sense, the Reformation refers to other movements within the Catholic Church, such as that of Calvin in Switzerland, which gave rise to the Evangelical Church, and that of Henry VIII in England, from which the Anglican Church emerged. These movements led to the Council of Trent, initiating a process of internal reform in the Catholic Church. Today, with the presence of Pope Francis, there is a move towards communion between these Churches.

In November 2016, Pope Francis extended to all priests the power to forgive the sin of abortion, which had only been delegated to bishops on a temporary basis. Forgiveness had already been authorized for all Catholic priests during the Year of Mercy, which ended on November 20. In the apostolic letter *Misericordia et Misera*, which deals with this authorization, Pope Francis makes it clear that this right will remain a new reality of his papacy." *I want to reiterate with all my might that abortion is a grave sin, because it puts an end to an innocent life, but with equal force, I can and must verify that there is no sin that God's mercy cannot reach and destroy when it finds a repentant heart that asks to be reconciled with the Father. Therefore, every priest should guide, support and comfort the penitents on this path of special reconciliation,"* he wrote.

"In order that there may be no obstacle between the request for reconciliation and God's forgiveness, I now grant all priests, by virtue of their ministry, the power to absolve all persons who have committed the sin of abortion. "

According to Catholic doctrine, abortion is a grave sin punishable by automatic excommunication of those involved. Forgiveness can only be given by those who have been delegated by the Pope after confession and repentance.

In his exhortation the Pope deals with abortion: *"No right to one's own body can justify a decision to end life".*

Forgiveness does not remove the sin of abortion from Catholic doctrine

When it comes to analyzing abortion from a religious perspective, it is undoubtedly the view of the Catholic religion that is the first to be observed and that deserves the most attention. The Catholic Church is not the oldest, but it covers a period of approximately two thousand years and recounts the events of one of the oldest religious institutions in activity, influencing the world in spiritual, religious, moral, political and socio-cultural aspects. The history of the Catholic Church is integral to the history of Christianity and the history of Western civilization.

According to its Catechism, "it is only with the eyes of faith that one can see its visible reality, which is at the same time a spiritual reality, the bearer of divine life."

The Catholic religion is held by the majority of the world's Latin American populations. Like others such as Anglican, Evangelical, Episcopalian, Protestant, whether Lutheran or Calvinist, and many other sects or doctrines that adopt Christianity, it considers that human beings have life from conception. The followers of this religion do not accept the fully liberalized practice of abortion, as they consider its practice to be the death of the unborn child. (10)

As for the unborn child, his or her life must be preserved from conception. (10) Therefore, for Catholics, life is inviolable from conception, that is, from the moment of fertilization, the union of the male spermatozoon with the female ovum.

Christianity predominates in the societies of the Western world, and the largest religion among those that venerate Jesus is Catholicism, which has its center in the Vatican State, making it the only religion that has a nation under its dominion: the Vatican, headed by the Pope.

Followers of Catholicism do not accept any reason for terminating a pregnancy, which makes them different from others who justify abortion at specific times.

Catholics believe that if they don't commit sins during their time on earth, they will be rewarded with eternal life in heaven.

To do this, Catholics must fulfill all the obligations of the Church's dogmas and doctrine.

The governments of predominantly Catholic countries consider themselves secular, i.e. they are not affiliated with religions and are opposed to ecclesiastics. In this sense, Dom Claudio Hummes, Cardinal Archbishop of Sao Paulo, Brazil, said: *"If it is true that the State is secular, it must not be forgotten that it is at the service of a people who have a religion and ethics. "* (9) Most Western countries call themselves secular, but not all have a position of allowing abortion to take place without any restrictions.

Unlike the Catholic religion, whose followers spread out without any concern for grouping together, the followers of the Jewish religion come together to practice mutual aid. This is how Jewish marriages usually take place between members of the same religion. It is common for Jewish settlements to have institutions such as hospitals for health care and schools for education, obeying religious precepts. Therefore, alongside traces of the cultures of the societies in which they live, followers of Judaism retain traces of the culture of their religion. Judaism considers that a fetus or embryo does not have the status of a person before birth. Within the Jewish population of the world, which can be considered an ethnic group, there are distinct ethnic divisions, most of which are the result of the geographical ramifications of the Israeli population, and subsequently of independent developments. Various Jewish communities have been established by Jewish settlers in many places around the world. (11)

Today, manifestations of these differences between Jewish ethnic divisions can be seen in the Jewish cultural expressions of each community, in Jewish linguistic diversity and in the mixtures between Jewish populations. Ethnic divisions among Jews have been divided into two main groups: Ashkenazis and Sephardim. These two groups are characterized by their place of residence. The Ashkenazis settled more in the Anglo-Germanic part of Europe. The Sephardim seek to live on the Latin side, while the Mizrahim and Teimanim or "Yemenites" are located in the eastern part of the world.

With regard to abortion in the Jewish religion, if the embryo or fetus poses a risk to the woman's health, abortion is permitted among the Orthodox, Conservative and Reform groups. (11) According to the tradition of Maimonides, in the 12th century, if the embryo endangers the woman's life, mental and physical health, she can terminate the pregnancy in self-defense, since the embryo would be considered an aggressor. However, the decision had to be made alongside a rabbi. (11) It is important to note that compared to Christianity, the traditionalism of the Jewish religion does not allow the termination of pregnancy to be an individual decision of the woman, but that this desire be accompanied by the permission of the rabbi who in his wisdom finds a moral and just reason. (11)

From a Buddhist point of view, abortion is considered murder. However, there can be various motivations for terminating a pregnancy. If the motivation is selfish unconcern, such as not wanting the obligation to look after a baby, this makes the act more serious in Buddhist eyes, because both the motivation and the act itself are destructive. (11) In Buddhism, the motivation can also be positive. If the baby is greatly deformed or mentally handicapped, then, wishing the child to avoid all future problems, abortion is not condemned because of the secondary bodhisattva vow taken by all Buddhists not to avoid committing a destructive action when the motivation is positive. However, the ethics of the problem are still questionable.

In another situation, in the case of risk to the mother during pregnancy, many circumstantial factors come into play when making a decision, and it is defined that the karma resulting from the decision will judge the individual in the next life depending on the circumstances of the abortion. In addition to causal motivations, Buddhist teachings dictate that contemporary motivation (what a certain individual thinks at the time of the abortion process) is also very important in justifying the act. Thus, it is very important for a Buddhist to have affectionate thoughts towards the baby at the time of the abortion. (11) Some Buddhist traditions perform ceremonies for the fetus. These ceremonies are supposed to be extremely helpful for the mother's "soul". The fetus is given a name and prays for its life. "The goal of Buddhists is to achieve spiritual improvement, "nirvana", a state of liberation from unhappiness and pain in the world, a spirituality of peace and happiness." Although there is no consensus within Buddhism on abortion, most of its followers consider it a breach of the precept not to take life. Traditional Buddhist sources, such as the Buddhist monastic code, point out that the deliberate destruction of life is a serious breach of precept. The current Dalai Lama considers abortion to be wrong, but believes that there are occasions that justify it. (**) Even when abortion is done to save a woman's life, it is almost always seen as causing suffering and negative karma. (**)

The followers of Islam, although the Heart condemns the act of killing, are very attached to a fanaticism about going to war, for example, in which they don't worry about dying, with the idea that death will bring them to the presence of Allah. In recent times, this fanaticism has affected a large number of young men, who often explode bombs affixed to their bodies in crowded places with the intention of committing acts of terrorism and without worrying about dying. The main cause of the condemnation of abortion among Muslims has historical roots. (11) The Bedouin peoples saw infanticide and abortion as a concern because of the need to have men to equip armies for the desired expansion in Africa, Asia and Europe. (11) The attitude of these terrorists is reprehensible, because it is carried out in wars of conquest, not least because the colonization of peoples by the Islamists was much more permissive than the European process in the Americas. (11) In the Islamist faith, on the last day of humanity, the children will be witnesses against the parents who killed them. (11) Most followers of Islam consider abortion permissible up to 120 days of gestation when the fetus or embryo has a life condition similar to animals or plants and for this reason this is the maximum limit for the practice of abortion regardless of the fact that leads to it.In the case of risk to the woman's life, for Islam it is preferable to save the primary life, that is, the life of the mother. If a pregnancy is accidentally terminated, compensation must be paid to the father because the life of an embryo is lost through the accident. The value of the life of an embryo is different from that of a fetus. If the pregnancy is terminated before the fifth month of pregnancy, 10% of the value of a life should be paid to the father; if it is terminated afterwards, the value is the total value of a life. (11) Abortion in Islam is permitted if there is an acceptable justification. There are, however, groups for whom termination of pregnancy is unacceptable.

Hinduism is a religion that contains several gods who are worshipped on different occasions and in different places. However, in a general sense, it classifies abortion as an abominable act. It is a kind of union of beliefs and lifestyles. Its religious culture is the union of ethnic traditions. It is currently the third largest religion in the world by number of followers. It originated around 3,000 AD in the ancient Vedic culture. Its followers respect ancient things and tradition, believe in sacred books, believe in deities, persist in the caste system, which determines the status of each person in society, know the importance of rites, trust spiritual guides and also believe in the existence of previous incarnations. A person's birth within a caste is the result of karma produced in past lives. Only the Brahmins, belonging to the "higher" castes, can perform Hindu religious rituals and assume positions of authority within the temples. (**) Among the gods, the main ones are: Brahma represents the creative force of the Universe, Ganesha goddess of wisdom and luck, Matsya who saved the human race from destruction, Sarasvati goddess of the arts and music, Shiva supreme god, creator of Yoga, Vishnu responsible for maintaining the Universe. (**).

The Church of Jesus Christ of Latter-day Saints, the Mormons, do not recommend abortions; on the contrary, they oppose them. However, if it is to preserve the woman's health or if the pregnancy is the result of rape, in this case to save the woman's spiritual health, the procedure is permitted by the President of the Church after consulting a doctor. The nickname Mormons was created by people who did not belong to the Church to refer to members of the Latter Day Saint movement. The name comes from a so-called sacred book of scripture compiled by the ancient prophet Mormon, entitled The Book of Mormon, Another Testament of Jesus Christ. According to the official version of the church, the name given by the Lord, by which the members of the Church are to be known, is Latter-day Saints. (**) According to the doctrine of the church, in this dispensation, which is that of the fullness of times or the last dispensation before the glorious day of the second coming of Jesus Christ, "Latter-day Saint" has been included to designate the members of the church at this time. The word Mormon actually originates from the Book of Mormon, a book compiled by the prophet Mormon, named after a place where King Noe's people lived and which, according to the prophet Joseph Smith himself, simply means "very good" (**).The Mormons have their main headquarters in the United States of North America where their first Church was formalized on April 6, 1830. The main center is located in Salt Lake City in the state of Utah. The Mormons spread throughout the world on missionary missions preaching Christianity and attracting new followers.

For followers of the Protestant Baptist, Lutheran, Presbyterian. Unitarian and Methodist churches, there is a wider range of attitudes towards abortion. In Protestant religious doctrine, there is a wider range of attitudes towards abortion than in the Catholic Church.

In a clarification, the Archbishop of Canterbury stated that *"For Church and State, the unity of moral respect and the human person. "*

Abbot Downside maintains that *"there is no determining moment, apart from the moment of conception, at which one can reasonably biologically and physiologically determine that human life begins. Nevertheless, I find it difficult to admit that it begins at that point. "*

The big difference between Catholics and most Protestant churches is respect for the life of the mother. Thus, everyone agrees that it is at the moment of conception that the mother acquires all the personal rights and entitlements of motherhood, since she is responsible for gestating, caring for and nurturing the embryo from the moment of its conception until the moment of its birth. At the same time, it must be seen that the doctor has a primary duty towards the mother, as she is the person who requested it. Therefore, if a choice has to be made between the life of the mother and that of the embryo or fetus, it will always be the mother who has priority, and it is therefore up to the doctor to decide, in the final analysis, when he can release the mother from her responsibility towards the fetus. Protestant countries were the first in this century to adopt more liberal legislation on abortion (**).

The Anglican Church is considered by many to be Catholic because it does not adopt heresies in its declarations of faith. But it is not "Roman", it is not subject to the pope, nor does it adopt his particular dogmas and practices: the transubstantiation of the elements of the Eucharist, prayer for the dead, obligatory celibacy of priests, veneration of the Virgin Mary and the canonized saints, the immaculate conception of Mary, the bodily assumption of Mary into heaven, the sacrifice of the Mass, purgatory, the infallibility of the pope, meritorious works for the salvation of the soul, tradition with the same value as the Holy Scriptures, and others.

As far as abortion is concerned, there is permission for it to take place, even though many followers of the Anglican Church are against it. (**)

The Methodists, through the Church's Episcopal College, sent a statement to the family that read as follows:

"The Episcopal College of the Methodist Church addresses the Methodist family on Brazilian soil to pass on its position on Bill number 1.135/91, regarding the interruption of pregnancy (abortion), which is currently before the National Congress.

We reaffirm it in the context of the Church's social doctrine:
a) Life is a gift from God (Genesis 1 and 2; Psalm 8); we believe in the Creator God!
b) The family community expresses fundamental requirements of God's creation.
c) The family is subject to economic insecurity and the tensions and maladjustments that accompany socio-cultural change.
d) Family planning is an essential factor, resulting in conscious parenthood, adjustment between spouses, the upbringing of children and home management.
e) The Methodist Church accepts and recommends the use of the resources of modern medicine for birth control, when it is not contrary to Christian ethics.
f) In Christian ethics, sex is considered a gift from God, the life he created.
g) Sex education is the responsibility of the family, the Church and educational institutions.
h) Sexual activity should be carried out responsibly and in the context of marriage, where love and commitment are present.
i) We believe in God's grace and, in this direction, we promulgate an ethic committed to the defense of life.
Regarding the issue of abortion, considering the postulates reported, the Methodist Church:

• It reaffirms its opposition to the practice of abortion, as well as its position that life is a gift from God and needs to be preserved and dignified from conception to death, in accordance with its statement in October 1986 at the National Congress of Women in Mariapolis, São Paulo. For this reason, it considers it extremely important to provide women with sexual education, a fair family income, access to birth control (not abortifacients) and dignified support for the wonderful act of "giving birth".
• It presupposes abortion in extreme cases, when the mother's life is at stake, because she must be able to have more children and must also have the chance to care for existing children who depend on her for their survival.
• Likewise, the possibility of abortion is allowed in cases of rape, if the woman so wishes, considering that she has not been given the chance to choose whether or not to have sex, which goes against the spirit of the Gospel proclaimed by our Lord Jesus Christ.
• Termination of pregnancy is allowed in cases where medicine proves that the fetus cannot survive, such as anencephaly (a fetus without an encephalic mass, which only remains alive as long as it is nourished by the mother's body).
The Methodist Church assumes an education for life. The defense of life includes a whole range of situations that need to be analyzed in the light of the gospel in terms of Jesus' message: "I have come that they may have life, and have it to the full" (Jodo 10.10).
The Episcopal College considers that the issue of "decriminalization of abortion", which is being discussed in the National Congress, is of the utmost importance and needs to be worked on both scientifically, ethically, morally, socially and from the point of view of public health, and always from the perspective of the ethics of the Gospel of Jesus Christ.
May the grace of the Lord Jesus Christ help us to walk forward, seeking to live out Jesus Christ's plan for the lives of our people.
Sao Paulo, June 5, 2007.
Bishop Joao Carlos Lopes - President of the Episcopal College
Bishop Luiz Vergilio Batista da Rosa - Vice-President of the Episcopal College Bishop Adonias Pereira do Lago - Secretary of the Episcopal College (**)

The splendid followers of Allan Kardec's book are against abortion even in cases where the woman has been the victim of rape. They believe that malformed fetuses should be born because they bring the parents a trial that they must go through in their lives

As for the beginning of life, they believe that the union begins at conception, but is not complete until birth. From the moment of conception, the Spirit assigned to inhabit a certain body is bound to it by a fluidic lake, which grows tighter and tighter until the moment the child sees the light. The cry that the newborn lets out announces that it is among the number of the living and the servants of God. (**)

The Universal Church of the Kingdom of God (Igreja Universal do Reino de Deus) is a neo-Pentecostal evangelical Christian denomination based in the Temple of Solomon in the city of Sao Paulo, Brazil. Founded on July 9, 1977 by Edir Macedo, it has become one of the largest neo-Pentecostal groups in Brazil. According to estimates, it has more than 6,000 temples, 12,000 pastors and 1.8 million faithful around the country. It has around 8 million followers and 15,000 pastors in 105 countries, and is most popular in Portuguese-speaking nations. It is one of the largest religious organizations in Brazil and the 29ª largest church in terms of followers in the world. (**)

In a public statement made more than ten years ago and recently reaffirmed, Pastor Macedo clarifies:

"I'm in favor of a woman's right to choose... I'm in favor of abortion, yes. The Bible is too... Look at this: 'If a man beget a hundred children, and live many years, even unto old age, and his soul be not filled with good things, and have no grave, I say that an abortion is happier than he. It's in Ecclesiastes, chapter 6, verse 3. Brazil should unite for a woman's right to choose abortion. Our leaders should strive for this and not bow down to pressure from certain religious segments. This would certainly reduce a large part of our social problems... Let's be cold and rational: is it better for the child not to come into the world or to see it in the garbage collecting food to survive? I believe in the Bible. In these cases, I believe that abortion is better than birth. A woman must have the right to choose. "

Macedo's position has become increasingly emphatic. Macedo has once again said: *"Yes, I'm in favor of abortion, and I'm saying it loud and clear, and if I'm sinning, I'm committing this conscious sin, yes!"*

The Jehovah's Witnesses are a Christian sect with followers in 240 countries and autonomous territories, with around 8 million practitioners, although they have a larger number of sympathizers. **0 are known for their regular and persistent preaching of their principles and dogmas from house to house, on the streets and in public places.

They worship exclusively the God presented in the Bible, calling him by the name Jehovah, and are followers of Jesus, having a different concept from other Christian groups who, for the most part, believe in the concept of a Triune God. They claim to biblically follow the instructions left by Jesus Christ, but reject the classification of being fundamentalists in the sense in which the term is commonly used. They seek to base all their practices and doctrines on the content of the Bible. Their organization is supported by financial donations from Jehovah's Witnesses around the world. Voluntary financial donations are important, but not vital, to maintain and expand the number of witnesses who dedicate their time to their educational work, respecting the laws of each country, having legal representation in which they are allowed and thus being legally instituted as a non-profit organization. (**)

As far as abortion is concerned, there is no definitive position, because if they consider that interrupting life is a grave sin and that the fetus is a living being, they accept what the societies in which they live have established as correct and legal regarding abortion.

Sex and sexual pleasure are accepted as desirable practices among those who follow Taoism and Confusionism. This practice should be observed with moderation, and should also be considered in relation to reproduction and abortion as an acceptable resource. However, groups of Taoists aiming to preserve life adopt views that are opposed to abortion. (**)

Many Native American cultures have a woman-centered view of reproductive issues, and abortion is a valid option.

Other existing religions do not have a large enough following to intervene in abortion, either by allowing it or restricting it.

9 Legislates and abortion

Although abortion is a procedure in which both the woman and the doctor are involved, neither the woman nor the doctor decides whether it can be performed. In reality, it is the tyrant in dictatorial governments or the parliament in democratic societies who decides whether this procedure is possible.

Abortion, whether spontaneous, induced, medicated or surgical, is an act that occurs in women and that requires medical attention in modern societies.

Society's decision to release or repress performance is based on various factors, including scientific ones.

The government's position on whether it considers itself secular or religious is the main factor, because if it adheres to a religion and that religion condemns the practice of abortion, there is nothing to be done. With regard to this statement, which may seem dubious at first, there is an illustrative example from the Catholic religion in the Vatican State. In Catholic doctrine, abortion is such a serious sin that those who perform it or suffer it are automatically excommunicated. Forgiveness for this sin lies solely in the hands of the Pope or whoever he delegates this act to. (**)

Societies dominated by tyrannies also take positions or impose restrictions preventing women from seeking medical attention even when they suffer a spontaneous abortion. El Salvador, a Central American country, condemns to death a woman who suffers an abortion for which she is unable to prove it was unprovoked. (**)

These examples are examples of what happens in the majority of countries which, if they don't totally free the possibility of abortion, don't totally repress it.

In most countries around the world, especially in the Western world, due to the varied composition of their parliaments, there is a mixture of proposed restrictions. Although they respond to concerns stemming from scientific knowledge, they are parliaments that, to a greater or lesser extent, translate popular opinions and exalt the values of the people to a greater or lesser extent. The values of medicine and the desires of women are heard and mixed with religious dogma, socio-economic conditions, the age composition of the population, the orientation of political parties and so many other factors that surround parliamentary decisions.

Thus, there are laws that fully allow abortion depending on the length of the pregnancy. Generally, from 12 weeks to 24 weeks gestation, abortion has no legal restrictions.

Other countries do not punish abortion when the pregnancy is the result of rape.

In many countries, incest is also considered sufficient for abortion to take place.

In many countries, a medical factor predominates, i.e. when the woman is at risk of death or when there is no other way of saving the pregnant woman's life, as a possibility that allows abortion to be carried out. An abnormality in the fetus, in the case of anencephalic or microcephalic fetuses, is also a medical factor.

These laws usually come from congresses or chambers of deputies, which often decide depending on the different situations that occur in the country. It should also be remembered that higher bodies such as supreme or superior courts have the power to establish reasons for not punishing those who have practiced abortions as criminals.

These specific situations in Brazilian legislation include the situation where there is no other way to save the woman's life and rape.

In an article published in the São Paulo press (23), Dom Odilo Scherer, Cardinal of São Paulo, weighs in on the subject. His words are as follows: *"Brazil still lacks specific legislation that values and protects human life before birth. The Brazilian Constitution enshrines the inviolable right to life, and in chapter five, item ten, recognizes that human life begins at conception; despite this, the violation of the right to life of unborn human beings is tolerated and even promoted by projects that intend to make abortion legal, either in a generalized way, or in a specific way, for specific situations'"*.

Gandra Martins (10), when dealing with the inviolability of the right to life, states that *"In two recent decisions, the Federal Supreme Court has relativized a fundamental right enshrined in the Constitution to such an extent that it has become the supreme positive legislator."* He was referring to one of the two recent decisions, which allowed the therapeutic anticipation of childbirth, i.e. abortion when the pregnant woman has an anencephalic fetus.

Two voices that deserve great respect and that reflect the thinking of the Catholic religion.

Catholic thinking deserves a lot of attention, but it is a dogmatic position that does not take into account the physical and social aspects that must be observed when enacting legislation.
for a country's population.

The issues involved are not few, as Dom Odilo (22) mentions: *"the comfort of the pregnant woman and her family, the frustration of the dreams that every mother has for the child she bears, the social burden of caring for people who are not totally autonomous... But above all, the decision to give life to a human being, who has had the misfortune to be affected in his brain development by causes absolutely beyond his responsibility, is at stake "*

Many other issues need to be considered when dealing with a country with a population of over 200 million inhabitants. Starting with the same consideration of religion. The Catholic religion is the one most followed in Brazil, but there is a reasonable percentage of practitioners of other religions who must be respected.

In *addition* to the religious question, the physical situation of the fetus must also be taken into account, a question that Dom Odilo once again addressed when he said: *"Furthermore, there is the problem of a reliable diagnosis for each case, because as far as we know, microcephaly cannot be reliably diagnosed before an advanced stage of pregnancy. "* (22)

The medical aspects of legislation are taken care of by doctors who have the most advanced knowledge of the sciences in the world. There can be error, and there can be deception, facts to which everyone is subject.

The problem of quality of life needs to be addressed, because people without a brain or with an affected brain do not have the ability to enjoy life as much as others. This affects the whole family and can damage family harmony.

Legislation must, however, take care of other relevant aspects such as quality of life from a social point of view. Although Brazilian legislation is restricted in allowing abortion, as it only allows it on two specific and special occasions: when rape occurs and when there is no other means of saving the pregnant woman's life; the Federal Supreme Court has already decided to allow abortion on occasions when the pregnant woman is carrying an anencephalic fetus and understands that it will promptly discuss pregnancies in which there is evidence of a fetus with microcephaly.

The social issues of women who, for various reasons, are unable to offer their children a full social life are not addressed in many countries that maintain restrictions on abortion.

Women without a partner, women abandoned by their partner, women whose partner does not recognize their paternity, women who, without their partner, cannot afford to keep the child, women thrown out of the house by their relatives, children who will not know their father and so many other moments when a woman does not want or does not have the possibility of having a child are social aspects that have led women and children to social discrimination that those who have abortions legally or illegally do not encounter.

Women who are punished for the inviolability of life that comes from the unproven dogmatic conception of some religions.

Like all legislation, norms and laws are produced and drafted by men who take care of aspects of human life from conception onwards, satisfying many, but not all.

Mistakes and errors are part of it.

10 Abortion as a crime

At different times and in different places, abortion is criminalized as a serious offence under the existing criminal code. Thus, in Malta
and in El Salvador, where its practice is absolutely forbidden and even carries the penalty of death. In other countries such as Scandinavia, the Netherlands and the United Kingdom, among many others, there are no obstacles to permission.

In Greek mythology, dating back to ancient times, there are references to its practice and recommendation. The practice of abortion has not always been recriminalized; it went unpunished if it did not result in harm to the health or death of the pregnant woman. A look at the legislation of the various nations of the world reveals different ways of dealing with the issue.

Brazil, on the other hand, having been colonized by Portugal, a Catholic country, ended up accepting the   concept
along with its growth and development.
that abortion is a wrong procedure. This practice was typified in the imperial penal code and continued to be considered a crime in the "Penal Code of the Republic" (**).

Since 1940, in the Brazilian Penal Code, the crime of abortion has been better characterized and given greater scope. The latter is still in force today.

Brazilian legislation considers abortion to be a crime prescribed in the Brazilian Penal Code.(3) The Code deals with it in its Special Part in Title I - Crimes Against Life in its Chapter I - Crimes Against the Person.

Article 124
Carrying out an abortion on herself or consenting to it being carried out by someone else:
Penalty - imprisonment from 1 (one) to 3 (three) years.

Article 125
Performing an abortion without the consent of the pregnant woman.
Penalty - imprisonment from 3 (three) to 10 (ten) years.

Article 126
Performing an abortion with the consent of the pregnant woman.
Penalty - imprisonment from 1 (one) to 4 (four) years.

Article 128
Abortion performed by a doctor is not punishable:
I- if there is no other way to save the pregnant woman's life;
II- if the pregnancy is the result of rape and the abortion is preceded by the consent of the pregnant woman or, when incapacitated, her legal representative.

Article 128(I) establishes that abortion is not punishable if there is no other means of saving the pregnant woman's life.

In the twentieth century, people in favor of abortion tried to legalize the practice, extending its permission to cases in which there was a risk to the health of the pregnant woman. It was no longer a confrontation between the life of the child and the life of the woman, but between the life of the child and the health of the woman, understood not in the sense of an absence of illness, but as a state of perfect physical, psychic and emotional well-being, as defined by the World Health Organization. (9) This interpretation, if accepted, would practically justify all the other conditions for abortion.

Subsection II establishes that there is no punishment if the pregnancy is the result of rape. Carnal intercourse with a woman incapable of understanding the fact or with a woman under the age of fourteen is considered rape.

Therefore, anyone who has an abortion, whether a doctor or not, is a criminal covered by various articles of the Penal Code, and the woman who consents to undergo an abortion is also a criminal.

The difference in sentence is not only in time but also in the severity of the sentence. A prison sentence must be served in a closed, semi-open or open regime. Detention must be served in a semi-open or open regime, unless there is a need for transfer to a closed regime. (Edited by Law no. 7.209, of 11.7.1984)

On April 30, the Federal Supreme Court published the ruling that allowed an anencephalic fetus to terminate its pregnancy. The judgment took place in April 2012. By eight votes to two, the majority of justices followed the vote of the rapporteur, Justice Marco Aurelio. In addition to the rapporteur, Justices Rosa Weber; Joaquim Barbosa; Luiz Fux; Carmen Lucia; Ayres Britto (retired); Gilmar Mendes; and Celso de Mello voted in favor of decriminalization. For seven of the ten ministers who took part in the judgment, it is not an abortion because there is no possibility of life for the fetus outside the womb. (**)

In the judgment, the ministers decided that doctors who perform the surgery and pregnant women who decide to terminate the pregnancy do not commit any kind of crime. With the decision, in order to terminate the pregnancy of an anencephalic fetus, women do not need a court decision authorizing them to do so. A diagnosis of anencephaly is enough. (**)

The criminal law, as set out in the current Brazilian Penal Code in the three articles that deal with abortion, shows right away that the desire is to punish rather than to ensure that abortion does not take place. Article 124 punishes a woman who has an abortion under any of the conditions laid down in article 128, i.e. if the abortion takes place because of rape or if there is no means of saving the pregnant woman's life. The exception is if the woman is pregnant with a fetus with anencephaly.

Articles 125 and 126 punish doctors who carry out abortions, excluding those carried out in accordance with Article 128 and the decision of the Supreme Court. The variation between these articles lies in the type of punishment, whether detention or imprisonment, and the length of time of loss of liberty.

Article 128 makes it clear that "abortion performed by a doctor is not punishable" if the pregnancy is the result of rape or if there are means to save the life of the pregnant woman. It is not punished, but the crime continues, unless the Supreme Court agrees that the fetus is anencephalic, when abortion is not considered a crime.

It's a mistake to believe that imprisoning the convict will solve the problem. Prevention work is needed.

The government should ensure that crime does not occur by analyzing the reasons that lead women to have an illegal abortion. Illegal, because all abortions are criminal.

To avoid abortion, it is necessary to avoid pregnancy.

How to avoid pregnancy: the need arises for young people from puberty onwards to know how pregnancy occurs and how to avoid it. The subject should be approached from the point of view of sexuality, showing how it occurs physiologically. It's a subject that could perfectly well be taught in secondary schools. Many girls go for a miscarriage because they got pregnant without knowing why they got pregnant.

Abortion is a public health problem and should be treated as such. As the city of Campinas in Sao Paulo has done, Br.(**)

Not with intense and periodic campaigns, but with a permanent program warning men and women to avoid pregnancy with all the existing methodology, from the Ogino and Knauss table to the use of different types of condoms, such as Condon for men and the IUD for women.

For the underprivileged, a sexual orientation service and the distribution of condoms should be set up in health centers or parallel activity institutes.

This program offers a double result, because in addition to preventing pregnancies in order to prevent abortions due to undesirable pregnancies, it would also achieve results as a family planning program.

So instead of giving away fish, people would be taught how to fish.

11 Final considerations

In society you will find many events related to abortion by coincidence, by chance and by so many other situations that demonstrate not only the frequency but also the importance of these events in scientific circles, social circles, political circles, religious circles, ethical circles, financial circles, family circles and others.

After looking at abortion from different perspectives and before closing the subject, it is possible to exemplify some of them that seem more disparate.

In Canada, although abortion is legal, eight nurses were dismissed from a hospital in Ontario for not agreeing to take part in the procedure. Unhappy with the hospital management's decision, they appealed to the Ontario Human Rights Commission, which decided that they should return to their jobs because, among other reasons, their contract of employment included a clause releasing them from the obligation to take part in such procedures. They returned and were no longer assigned to abortion practices. In many other places in different countries, the refusal to participate on the grounds of conscientious objection has led to the dismissal of professionals. Many of them appealed and were reinstated. (9)

The press in Sao Paulo, Brazil, has reported that a Catholic priest has been convicted by the Superior Court of Justice of interrupting a legal abortion. The case took place in the interior of Goias, a state in the center of the country. 11 years ago, the priest filed a writ of habeas corpus to prevent a pregnant woman from having an abortion of a fetus diagnosed with Body Stalk Syndrome - a set of malformations that make life outside the womb impossible. The woman was already in hospital, medicated and ready for surgery when she was forced to return home. She spent the next eight days in pain until, back at the hospital, a fetus was born and died immediately. Her parents then filed a lawsuit for moral damages, which was rejected by the Goias courts. Referred to the Superior Court of Justice, the appeal was upheld and the priest was ordered to pay sixty thousand reais - about twenty thousand dollars - for "seeking state protection to defend his private ideas about terminating a pregnancy" and that with his attitude he had attacked the rights of the mother and father who had the legal guarantee to terminate the pregnancy. The judge highlighted the Supreme Court's 2012 decision that ruled out the possibility of criminalizing the termination of anencephalic pregnancies.

In Rio de Janeiro, the Curia of the Archdiocese disallowed the support of religious for Marcelo Freixo, the 2016 candidate for mayor of the city supported by movements of the political left.(21) Ten priests, a friar and a nun and more than 800 lay people published a text saying that Freijo's candidacy was in line with the preaching of Pope Francis. The Archdiocese was perplexed and condemned the move, arguing that the aforementioned candidate was in favour of decriminalizing abortion and same-sex unions.

The Court of Justice of Sao Paulo. A twenty-three year old housewife, seven months pregnant, was refused an abortion because the fetus had hydrocephalus. The pregnant woman appealed and the president of the Superior Court of Justice of Sao

Paulo modified the first two decisions and in the third instance authorized the abortion of the child with hydrocephalus in Brazil. (9)

In France, a woman named Josette Perruche was pregnant when her eldest daughter contracted rubeola. She went for a medical examination in order to have an abortion if she was infected with the rubeola virus. The test came back negative. Josette carried the pregnancy to term and gave birth to Nicolas, who was born with various rubeola-related disorders such as deafness, heart disease and neurological problems. Ten years later, in 1992, Nicolas' parents filed a lawsuit against the doctor who carried out the negative test and won the case. They later appealed on behalf of their son Nicolas. They asked in a surreal way for him to be compensated for having been born. The French Supreme Court accepted the request and ruled that "since the doctors prevented Josette from terminating the pregnancy in order to avoid the birth of a disabled child, she can sue and receive compensation for the medical error." The newspaper Le Monde challenged the ruling with an editorial in which it asked whether life itself could constitute damage that gives rise to a right to compensation.(9)

In Brazil, in Sao Paulo, a medical journal reports a fact that contradicts those who consider that a woman who undergoes an abortion
suffers psychological problems. This is the case of a girl under thirteen who was raped by two men during a funk dance. As a result of the rape, the girl became pregnant and was three months pregnant when she was taken to the doctor. The girl wanted an abortion because she was repulsed by the child. The religious mother and the doctor, who was also religious, didn't agree and forced the pregnancy to end. Years passed and the child, who was already six years old, began to go with her mother to a Home for Adolescents, where she and her grandmother were treated by psychologists, because her nineteen-year-old mother didn't recognize her daughter. The mother of the girl who became pregnant, i.e. the grandmother of the six-year-old girl, does not accept the situation. As a consequence of not having an abortion, family life is terrible.

A 34-year-old engineer became a widower two years ago. His wife died at the age of 30 as a result of complications from an illegal abortion carried out in a clandestine clinic in Recife, Pernambuco, Brazil. Because she didn't want the child and her husband was traveling, she went to a clinic to have an abortion. Due to perforation of the uterus and other organs as a result of an error on the part of the doctor performing the operation, she was rushed to a private hospital. Her husband, who was informed of the event, said: "My wife didn't just die. She was murdered." Statements like this are found in the press and are a product of the legal impossibility of performing abortion in safe conditions with competent doctors.

In many parts of the world, the discussion about the decision to have an abortion, as has already been mentioned, is beyond the control of the woman and the doctor.

In the United States of America, a country with a Catholic minority, several politicians differ with the religious authorities on the abortion controversy. Such was the case between Bill Clinton and Pope John Paul II in 1998, when they had many disagreements.(9)

In the last debate before the election period between Hillary Clinton and Donald Trump, candidates for the presidency of the United States of America, the subject came up, showing the voters' interest in knowing the two candidates' opinions on abortion.

Donald Trump in one of his first statements after being elected President of the United States of America in November 2016 revealed his desire to repeal US legislation on abortion in force since 1973.

The Republican congressional caucus, the ones that supported Trump, immediately after the new president's inauguration declared that they will try to modify the abortion legislation proposed by President Obama's administration.

George W. Bush, President of the United States of America, always had the support of the population groups that were against allowing abortion. Both Al Gore and John Kerry in 2000 and 2004 would have had a better chance of defeating George Bush if they hadn't come out in favor of abortion. The New York Time, a prestigious newspaper in the United States, reported that George Bush won the election because of his views on abortion. (9)

Political speeches are always made at times of personal interest when the subject is under discussion and the politician wants to reach a significant audience. Orestes Quercia, candidate for Governor of the State of São Paulo in 1986, when asked about abortion, replied: "As a man, I am completely opposed to abortion for ethical and even religious reasons, but as a politician it is a problem that is there." (9)

Geraldo Alckmim, when he was running for mayor of São Paulo, said that "abortion is not a solution". Six years later, as a candidate for the Presidency of the Republic, he declared that he was in favor of abortion in cases where the Brazilian Penal Code does not punish abortion, rape and there is no other way to save the life of the pregnant woman.(9)

In 1995, federal deputy Jose Genuino presented a bill authorizing abortion in the first ninety days of pregnancy, at the woman's free request. Discussed in the Chamber of Deputies, the bill was rejected by politicians without considering medical reasons. (9)

The following year, Congresswoman Marta Suplicy presented a bill to free abortion in the case of fetal malformations. She abandoned the bill because she was running for mayor of Sao Paulo. These two representatives of Sao Paulo in the
The National Congress has tried on several occasions to table motions to liberalize the abortion procedure. (9)

In the 1998 election campaign in which Fernando Henrique Cardoso was elected President of Brazil, the issue of abortion was discussed by the candidates. In that campaign, the losing candidate Ciro Gomes told the press that it was impossible to ignore the serious social problem that allowed rich women to have abortions in the best possible hygienic conditions and poor women in the worst. Society is hypocritical in that rich, white women are admitted to hospitals and poor, black women are forced to have abortions themselves. He promised to put an end to hypocrisy. (9)

In 2000, Luiza Erundina, candidate for mayor of Sao Paulo, declared herself in favor of abortion, but that she would never undergo the procedure.

With the start of the 2002 presidential election campaign, the candidates were asked about abortion. Anthony Garotinho, Governor of Rio de Janeiro, an avowed evangelical, said in a television interview that he was against abortion and euthanasia.

Jose Serra, candidate for the Presidency of the Republic of Brazil in 2002, declared that he foresaw carnage if abortion were legalized.

More than once, Lula, a candidate for the Presidency of the Republic of Brazil, claimed that there were more than two million clandestine abortions in Brazil, without having any way of proving it. (9)

In 2006, Jandira Feghali, the favorite candidate for Senator for the state of Rio de Janeiro, lost her election when she tried, in a timely manner, to prevent the Catholic Church from criticizing her position in favor of abortion. (9)

Bishop of the Universal Church of the Kingdom of God founded in Brazil and candidate for mayor of the city of Rio de Janeiro, Marcelo Crivella said in a 2012 sermon, according to newspaper reports, that homosexuality could still originate in the mother's womb, the result of a botched abortion.

These and so many other examples show that the problem of abortion is distanced from the important members of its practice, the woman and the doctor, finally reaching a dilemma with a high level of participation by politicians who care more about their careers and their popularity and make decisions to free abortion or prevent it from taking place. Often, not even religious, ethical, social, economic, population or health considerations are taken into account.

This subject is treated in a way that is far removed from the scientific knowledge of medicine, yet it is considered to be the most frequent episode that occurs in obstetrics. However, the results of polls, surveys, opinions and other ways of obtaining data from the darkness that hides the reality of abortions do not allow us to clearly understand their incidence.

There is an estimate, albeit modest, that when Brazilian women reach the end of their reproductive life, around the age of 50, one in five has had an abortion. This is a percentage of 20%, which is lower than the results presented in previous quotes. The Hospital Universitario de Santa Maria in Rio Grande do Sul, which has some of the most advanced care in the country, considers that an average of 15 to 20% of pregnant women miscarry. Another medical school, the Federal University of Sao Paulo, agrees with this estimate. (**) The studies shown in the previous chapter arrive at higher figures, but for the sake of prudence it is better to establish lower figures.

The Brazilian press reports that four women die every day in hospitals from complications of abortion, most of which are carried out illegally.

This result leads to concern and a search for the causes that led to it and how to transform this darkness into a clear area in which the health sciences can act freely. This uncertainty about abortion means that society as a whole immediately sees two antagonistic positions on abortion.

These two positions contradict each other when it comes to discussing who should ethically decide on abortion. Those in favor of abortion cling to the woman's right to decide, because they claim that it is the woman who houses in her body the cells that make up the biological being she has generated, i.e. the fetus.

The naysayers, based on the woman's inability to decide about the fetus, because from conception the fetus is another living being.

A woman's autonomy includes her own decision, the right to freedom, privacy, personal choice and the possibility of following her own wishes by choosing her own course of action. This autonomy is limited when it comes up against the autonomy of another human being. This aspect is raised by those who deny the possibility of abortion, because the fetus, from the moment of fertilization, is, in the understanding of this group, another human being. They defend heteronomy. This brings us back to the dilemma of whether life is inviolable and sacred and when this condition should prevail, at conception or at birth.

This attitude of accepting the pregnant woman's choice and desire, provided she is responsible and has been clearly informed of all the consequences of her act, is reinforced if the dictates of beneficence and justice are obeyed. Undoubtedly, performed outside the shadows of illegality, as a clear and transparent attitude, abortion will not only comply with much more appropriate scientific standards, but the impact of guilt, of the hidden performance, will be overcome. Therefore, not only will a greater evil be avoided, but we will be acting in much better conditions for the woman's good. On the other hand, it is fair, because it will universalize the conditions, putting an end to the discrimination that takes place between women from better financial backgrounds and women who cannot afford to perform this act, who are subjected to undergoing it where it is generally carried out in inadequate conditions and with personnel who are partners in the violation of the law.

Permission to perform an abortion at the request of a pregnant woman does not oblige her to do so, but only allows those who wish to do so the opportunity to do so.

The freedom to have an abortion on the grounds of the woman's desire, or in defense of the woman's health, or on the grounds of her condition in relation to her family and society, with the consent or not of her partner, whether formal or fortuitous, and regardless of any justification other than the one she establishes for herself, is supported by the autonomy that all responsible and competent human beings possess and have the right to exercise.

What we don't want to do is prevent women or doctors from realizing their desires in complete freedom, in accordance with their consciences and religious devotions, without having to do so in the shadows,

The woman, who is responsible, aware and clearly informed of the risks she faces in having an abortion, will decide in a clear and transparent manner.

Luiz Garcez Leme, Professor of Geriatrics at the Faculty of Medicine of the University of Sao Paulo, said that if abortion were approved, "the state would have to hire professionals other than doctors, because 'we' doctors are not meant for this. Our commitment is to life." (9).

Finally, we need to understand that no woman is obliged to undergo an abortion and no doctor is obliged to carry it out if she doesn't want to.

References:

(1) Holy Bible. Old Testament. Pentateuch. Genesis I. The origins. -

(2) BBC Brazil. Abortion gains ground in several countries October 7, 2010.

(3) Brazilian Penal Code. Special Part, Title I Crimes against the person. Chapter I Crimes against life: Art.124, Art.125, Art.126, Art.127, Art.128. Special Part, Title VI Crimes against sexual dignity. Chapter I Crimes against sexual dignity: Art.213, Art.217.

(4) Federal Council of Medicine. Resolution No. 1811 of December 14, 2006.

(5) Federal Council of Medicine. Resolution No. 1989 of May 14, 2012.

(6) Federal Council of Medicine.1st National Meeting of Medical Councils, 2013

(7) Diniz, D. & Medeiros, M. Aborto no Brasil: uma pesquisa domiciliar com tecnica de urna. National Abortion Survey. Institute of Bioethics and Human Rights, Brasilia, 2010

(8) Engelhard, H.T. Fundamentos da Bioetica, translated by Jose A. Ceschin Editora Loyola, Sao Paulo, 1998.

(9) Martins, I.G.S. Martins, R.V.S. Martins Filho I.G.S. A Questao do Aborto: aspectos juridicos fundamentais, Sao Paulo, Quartier Latin, 2008.

(10) Martins,I.G.S.& Carvalho,P.B. (coord) Inviolability of the Right to Life, Sao Paulo, Noeses. 2013.

(11) Marques,A.C & Monteiro,P. Transatlantico do Conhecimento, Google, December 27, 2010.

(12) Meira, A.R. Society and Health, Center for Biological and Health Sciences, Federal University of Mato Grosso do Sul, Campo Grande, 1997.

(13) Meira, A.R. Contribuigao para o estudo da fertilidade na Cidade de Santos, Brasil in Revista Iatros,IV (1): 21-24 1° semestre/1985.

(14) Meira, A,R, & Ferraz,F.R.C. Liberagao do Aborto: opinião de estudantes de medicina e de direito. Sao Paulo, Brazil. Rev.Saude publ.S.Paulo, 23 (6) 46572,1989.

(15) Meira, A.R. Folhas Soltas: bioetica e meditagoes. Scortecci Editora, Sao Paulo, 2007.

(16) Meira, A.R. Abortion: opinion of medical academics. 27th Brazilian Congress of Human Reproduction. Sao Paulo, November 4, 2016.

(17) Meira, A.R. Abortamento: reflexoes Reprodugao e Climaterio 30 (2) 51-53,2015. Available at http:ZZdx.doi.org/10.1016Zj.recli.2015.09.003

(18) Monteiro,M.F.G. Adesse,L. Drezzet,J. Update of estimates of the magnitude of induced abortion, rates per thousand women and ratios per 100 live births of induced abortion by age group and major regions.Brazil,1995 to 2013. Reproduction and Climacteric 30 (1) 11-18,2015.

(19) Moura,R,M, Senado contra aborto para gravida com Zika, Metropole in O Estado de Sao Paulo pg A18, September 10, 2016.

(20) World Health Organization. Safe abortion: technical and policy guidance for health systems, 2nd ed. Translated into Portuguese by Silvia Pineyro Trias, Grafica S.A.

(21) Pennafort,R. Curia disallows religious support for Freixo.O Estado de S.Paulo Politica pg A9 October 27, 2016.

(22) Scherer, Dom Odilo P. Reasons in favor of abortion. The State of São Paulo A2 Espago Aberto, April 13, 2013.

(23) Scherer, Dom Odilo P. Statute of the Unborn - what's the problem? O Estado de S.Paulo A2 Espago Aberto, October 8, 2015.

(24) Scherer, Dom Odilo P. Abortion-some uncomfortable reflections. O Estado de S.Paulo A2 Espago Aberto, December 10, 2016.

(25) Torres,J.H.R. Aborto e a Legislagao Comparada, in Aborto Artigos, Sao Paulo, 2016.

(**) Information obtained from Google on the Internet.

The Author

Born in Sao Paulo on March 27, 1931, to Renato Meira and Gaetana Domemica Chiara Italia Splendore.

The maternal grandson of Alfonso Splendore, Professor of Medicine in Italy and author of valuable scientific works in Brazil on Toxoplasmosis, Blastomycosis, Sporotrichosis and on the eradication of the arvicole wheat parasite in Italy during World War I, which earned him the title of Commander of the Kingdom.

During his high school years at the Liceu Pasteur in Sao Paulo, which ended in 1948, he founded and edited a short-lived neighborhood newspaper called "O Bandeirante."

He graduated in medicine from the Escola Paulista de Medicina in 1955. He took a postgraduate course in Sociology and Anthropology in 1963/64 at the Postgraduate School of Social Sciences of the Sao Paulo School of Sociology and Politics. He obtained his doctorate in competitions held at the Faculty of Dentistry in 1965 and the Faculty of Medicine in 1976, both at the University of São Paulo. He was awarded the title of Full Professor in competitions held at the Faculty of Medical Sciences of Santos in 1974 and the Faculty of Medicine of the University of São Paulo in 1976, and was awarded the title of Full Professor of the Faculty of Medicine of the University of São Paulo in the Department of Legal Medicine, Medical Ethics and Social and Occupational Medicine in 1990.

He was Professor of Community Health at the Faculty of Medical Sciences of Santos from 1970/1987 and at the Faculty of Medicine of the ABC Foundation from 1972/1987 and Professor of Legal Medicine and Ethics at the Santo Amaro Faculty of Medicine from 1983/1987.

In his teaching and research career, he had the opportunity to collaborate with the University of Brasilia when it was planning and implementing the School of Medicine. He was Director of the Faculty of Medical Sciences of Santos from 1971 to 1973, as well as Director of the Faculty of Medicine of Santo Amaro in 1987. In 1982 he was Technical Assistant to the Rector of the University of São Paulo. As one of only three Brazilian professors to be awarded the status of Milbank Faculty Fellow, he undertook his Post-Doctoral Fellowship in 1968/69 at the University of Kentucky Medical School in the United States of America. In 1972, he was a Visiting Professor at the University of Nottingham in England. He taught ethics at the Escuela Latino Americana de Bioetica in Buenos Aires in 1990. From 1993 to 1995 he was Chief of Staff to the Superintendent of the Hospital das Clinicas de Sao Paulo.

Author of two bulletins, eight books, organizer and co-author of three others, he has collaborated with chapters in sixteen others, published in Brazil and abroad.

He has given courses and lectures in Brazil and in countries in the Americas, Europe and Asia.

He was the creator of the Cultural Bulletin of the Sao Paulo Academy of Medicine "Asclepio" and its editor from 2009 to 2011 and of the part corresponding to the Sao Paulo Academy of Medicine in the magazine "Inovar saude" until 2015. He is a member of the Cultural Council of the "Suplemento Cultural" (Cultural Supplement) of the Revista da Associagao Paulista de Medicina, where he frequently publishes articles.

He has published more than a hundred articles in magazines and specialized journals both in Brazil and abroad, as well as articles in the newspapers "O Estado de S.Paulo" "Diario Latino" in "Gazeta de Pinheiros" and commentaries in the Revista do Jockey Club de Sao Paulo.

He was awarded the 1961 Society of Legal Medicine and Criminology Prize and the 1988 Funda Centro Prize. He was honored as "Vult of Brazilian Legal Medicine" in 1990 at the II Brazilian Congress of Medical Ethics held in Florianopolis. In 1994, he was awarded the "Order of Sao-Pauline Perseverance"; in 2004, the "Medal of the Civil Order of the Noble Knights of Sao Paulo"; in 2007, the "Medal of Cultural Merit of the Brazilian Academy of Art, Culture and History"; and in the same year, he was named "Man of the Year" in a tribute paid to him by the Legislative Assembly of the State of Sao Paulo. In 2013, he was named "Man of Success" by ApparEnza magazine. He was honored with the Golden Jubilee of the Sovereign International Order of Sports Merit in 2014.

He joined the Sao Paulo Academy of Medicine in 1986, of which he is a Full Member Emeritus, of Chair No. 5 whose patron is Professor Doctor Alfonso Splendore, having participated as Director Treasurer 2009/2011 and President 2011/13 and 2013/2015.

Since 1989, his academic interests have focused on bioethics. He was one of the introducers of bioethics in his country. He was part of the organizing committee of the Latin American Federation of Bioethics Institutions, and was its first Vice President. He was the founder and President of the Brazilian Association of Medical Ethics for seven years and a founding member of the Brazilian Society of Bioethics (SBB). He chaired the II Brazilian Congress of Medical Ethics, held in Florianopolis in 1990. In 1994, he received a Gold Medal for his outstanding services to the Hospital das Clinicas of the Faculty of Medicine of the University of São Paulo. He organized and chaired the 1st Bioethics Congress of Latin America and the Caribbean, held in Sao Paulo in 1995.

He joined the Universidade Catolica de Santos in the "strictu sensu" Postgraduate Program in Public Health in 2001/03, as a lecturer in the subject Health, Society and Bioethics.

In 2004 he was awarded the title of Professor Emeritus by the Congregation of the Faculty of Medicine of the University of Sao Paulo.

Coordinator of specialization courses in Occupational Medicine, Forensic Medicine and Geriatrics offered by the Londrina Institute of Technology and Economic and Social Development, which were held at the Universidade do Oeste Paulista in Presidente Prudente from 2003 to 2010.

Coordinator of the Bioethics Committee of the Brazilian Society of Human Reproduction 2006-2008.

In 2007, he was elected to the Board of Directors of the APE - Associate of Emeritus Professors of the USP Faculty of Medicine.

Although he had a penchant for literature since high school, he founded a newspaper, "O Bandeirante", and published chronicles in another, "Diario Latino", which he continued during his youth when he periodically published health-related issues in both "Gazeta de Pinheiros" and "O Estado de S. Paulo", his literary inclinations began to emerge more vigorously in 2009, when he began to write poems. Praised and enthused by family members, his first poems were published in "Encontro casual", an anthology published by Editora Scortecci. Since then, he has been writing poems with greater or lesser intensity until the present day. His output in this field can be found in a book entitled "Nao Sou Poeta: sou fazedor de rimas" (I'm not a poet: I'm a rhymesmith), which really reflects what he considers himself to be. Finally, in a book that mixes his scientific training with his penchant for literature, he spontaneously recounts the most important aspects of his professional life. Published in 2016 under the title "Sixty years on, stories of a non-specialist doctor", the author explains why he wrote the book:

"The reason for this book is that when people ask me what I do for a living, I say:
- I'm a doctor.
Which produces the common question:
- What is your specialty?
I'll answer again with complete peace of mind:
- I'm a doctor, I trained as a doctor and not as a specialist."

The reason is found at the beginning of the book, while the rest of the book contains passages from his professional life as a general practitioner, anaesthetist, including the use of hypnotism to anaesthetize surgeries; laboratory scientist; expert in forensic medicine and medical ethics; sanitarian and professor and director of medical schools.

A keen sportsman, particularly soccer, he is dedicated to community life at Sao Paulo Futebol Clube, where he is a member of the Deliberative Council and the Advisory Council, President of the Deliberative Council (2004-2006), the club's sovereign body. In the 2006-2012 term, he was General Secretary, a position he held from 2000-2002. He is currently General Secretary of the Advisory Council.

As an oil painting enthusiast, he sometimes filled canvases, mainly with seascapes, which were shown in low-profile exhibitions.

Racehorse breeder and owner of Haras Kentucky, he was Director of the Sao Paulo Jockey Club for more than a dozen years.

For the last forty-two years he has shared all his moments of joy and sadness with Jugary de Barros.

He has two children from his first marriage: Mario Renato (who died in a car accident in 1990 at the age of 31); Silvia (born in 1961, with a PhD in Art History from the Sorbonne in Paris). Silvia has two sons, Douglas (born in 1994) and Rodolpho (born in 1999). Silvia is a Lecturer in Art History at the University of Sao Paulo.

Academic Titles

Medical degree from the Paulista School of Medicine (1955)
Specialist in the 1st Course in Nutrition and Public Health as a World Health
Organization Fellow.(1963)
Postgraduate degree in Social Sciences (Anthropology and Sociology) from the Sao
Paulo School of Sociology and Politics (1963/64).
PhD from the University of Sao Paulo (1965)
Full member of the Brazilian Society of Human Reproduction.
Founding Member of the Brazilian Society of Bioethics.
Assistant Doctor of Hygiene and Legal Dentistry, Faculty of Dentistry, University of
Sao Paulo (1955/65)
Oscar Freire Award from the Society of Legal Medicine and Criminology (1961)
French Government Fellow at the Faculte de Sciences, Sourbone, Paris (1996)
Associate Professor of Medical Anthropology, Faculty of Medicine, University of
Brasilia (1966/70)
Milbank Faculty Fellow (1967/72)
Post Doctoral Fellowship, University of Kentucky Medical School (1968/69)
Assistant Professor, Department of Community Health, Faculty of Medicine,
University of Sao Paulo (1970/76)
Professor of Community Health at the Faculty of Medical Sciences of Santos
(1970/87)
Professor of Community Health at the ABC Medical School (1972/87)
Professor of Community Health and Legal Medicine and Medical Ethics at the Santo
Amaro Dental and Medical Faculties (1978/87) Technical Assistant to the Rector of
the University of Sao Paulo (1980/82)
Fundacentro Award from the Occupational Medicine Foundation (1988)
Professor of Legal Medicine, Medical Ethics and Social and Occupational Medicine
at the Faculty of Medicine of the University of São Paulo (1976/90) President of the II
Brazilian Congress of Medical Ethics, Florianopolis (1990)
Full Professor of Legal Medicine, Medical Ethics and Social and Occupational
Medicine at the Faculty of Medicine of the University of Sao Paulo. (1990/93)
President of the 1st Congress of Bioethics of Latin America and the Caribbean Sao
Paulo. (1995)
Professor of Public Health at Universidade Catolica de Santos (2000/02)
Coordinator of specialization courses in Geriatrics, Legal Medicine and Occupational
Medicine, Universidade do Oeste Paulista (2002/10)
Professor Emeritus, Department of Legal Medicine, Medical Ethics and Social and
Occupational Medicine, Faculty of Medicine, University of Sao Paulo (2004)
President of the Sao Paulo Academy of Medicine (2011/2015)

Books and book chapters published.

Contribution to the series of tonsillectomies *performed under hypnotic anesthesia,* in collaboration with Candido Carrei, chapter 19, in A.C. de Moraes Passos and Oscar Farina **Aspectos actuais da Hipnologia** Linografica Editora Limitada, Sao Paulo, 1961.

Hypnosis in Dentistry: Legal Aspects and Hypnosis Regulation Project chapter 45 in A.C.de Morais Passos and Oscar Farina **Aspectos actuais da Hipnologia** Linografica Editora Limitada, Sao Paulo, 1961.

Hypnosis in medicine and law, Linografica Editora Ltda. Sao Paulo, 1963, pgs .85.

Sobradinho 66: levantamento geral da 5° regiao administrativa do Distrito Federal, Universidade de Brasilia, Faculdade de Ciencias Medicas, Distrito Federal, 1966, pgs. 20.

Health begins at home, A.R. Editora, Sao Paulo, 1973, p. 32.

Saude da Comunidade: temas de medicina preventiva e social (org) McGraw-Hill do Brasil, Sao Paulo, 1976, pgs. 295.

Health and disease pgs.1 to 5; *The doctor in the community: the medical subculture* (in col.) pgs.7 /12; *Epidemiology as a process of studying health problems in communities* pgs.87 /95 in Pareta,J.M.; Meira,A.R. and d'Andretta Jr.C. (orgs.) **Saude da Comunidade:temas de medicina preventiva e social**,McGraw-Hill do Brasil,Sao Paulo,1976, pgs.295.

Culture and specialization pgs. 355/359 in Interlandi,S.(org.) **Ortodontia**,Artes Medicas, Editora da Universidade de Sao Paulo,Sao Paulo,1977, pgs.364.

Aspectos medico-sociais pgs. 338 / 340 in Serro Azul,L.G. C.C..; Carvalho Filho,E.T. e Decourt,L.V. (orgs.) **Clfnica do individuo idoso**,Guanabara Koogan,Rio de Janeiro,1981, pgs.345.

Nogoes de Planejamento familiar e do controle da natalidade (org) Servigos de Artes Graficas da Coordenadoria de Atividades Culturais da Universidade de Sao Paulo, Sao Paulo, 1982, pgs.128.

Introduction-definitions pgs.13 /20; *Introduction to contraceptive methods* (in col.) pgs 71/76; Ethical and legal aspects of birth control 75 natalidade pgs.121/128- in Meira,A.R.(org.) **NoCoes de planejamento familiar e do controle da natalidade**,ServiCos de Artes Graficas da Coordenadoria de Atividades Culturais da Universidade de Sao Paulo,Sao Paulo,1982, pgs. 128.

Compendio de Medicina Legal (org) Sao Paulo,Saraiva,1987,,pgs. 377.

Aspectos legais e gravidez pgs.129 /133 in Zugaib,M. e Sancovski,M.(org.) **Pre-natal**, Livraria Ateneu Editora,Sao Paulo,1991, pgs. 133.

A sociedade e a saude: uma introduCao às noCoes de ciencias sociais aplicadas a saude, Universidade Federal de Mato Grosso do Sul ,Campo Grande,1997, pgs.103.

Culture and specialization pgs. 1/8 in Interlandi,S.(org.) **Ortodontia** 4 edigao, modificada, ampliada e atualizada,Artes Medicas,Sao Paulo,1999, pgs. 769.

The health professional, culture and bioethics pgs.11/25 in Pinto,R.M.F.e Silva,W.V. (eds)**Temas de Saude Publica: qualidade de vida**, Leopoldianum,Santos, 2001, pgs. 235.

Ears in Sampaio,G.S. **Estoria de um Mangalarga** Sao Paulo,Scortecci, 2002, pgs. 114.

Evolugdo:assunto a discutir pgs 261/260 in Neves,M.C.P, e Lima,M (Org) in **Bioetica ou Bioeticas: na evolugao das sociedades**,Edigao Luso-Brasileira,Grafica de Coimbra 2 e Centro Universitario Sao Camilo,Coimbra, 2005, pgs.387.

Loose Leaves: bioethics and meditations. Scortecci Publishing Group. Sao Paulo, 2007, pgs.308.

Incendio na floresta and Terra dos Passaros (poems) pgs. 9/13 in **Encontro Pontual** anthology Grupo Editorial Scortecci, Sao Paulo, 2010, pgs. 366.

I'm not a poet: I make rhymes. Grupo Editorial Scortecci.Sao Paulo, 2010, pgs. 116.

Code of Medical Ethics: comparisons and reflections. Grupo Editorial Scortecci.Sao Paulo, 2010, pgs. 192.

Affonso Renato Meira pgs. 133/169 in Martins,I.G.S. e Bastos Neto,J.A.(coord) **Rimas Tricolores:poesias e cronicas.** Giordanus for Pax & Spes. Sao Paulo, 2011, pgs. 294.

Department of Legal Medicine, Medical Ethics and Social and Occupational Medicine (in coll.) pgs.108/123 in Mota,A and Marinho,M.G.S.M.C.(org) **Departamentos da Faculdade de Medicina da Universidade de Sao Paulo:Memorias e Historias.** Sao Paulo:CD.G Casa de Solugoes e Editora, 2012,pgs. 285.

7 de margo (org) Sao Paulo: Academia de Medicina de Sao Paulo, 2012, pgs. 308

Introduction pgs. 01/04 in Meira,A.R. Palomba, G.A. Helio Begliomini in **7 de margo,** Meira,A.R.,Palomba, G.A.Begliomini,H. Sao Paulo Academy of Medicine, Sao Paulo, 2012, pgs. 308.

Affonso Renato Meira pgs.28 to 30 in Meira, A.R. Palomba, G.A. e Begliomini,H. in **7 de margo** Academia de Medicina de Sao Paulo,Sao Paulo, 2012, pgs. 308.

Affonso Renato Meira pgs.23/38 in Padilha,E.S. **Os 14 Cardeais do** Sao **Paulo Futebol Clube** Sao Paulo: Scorrtecci, 2014, pgs. 217.

Alfonso Splendore pgs 38/40 in Begliomini,H. **Progonos da Academia de Medicina de Sao Paulo,** Sao Paulo, Expressao & Artes Editora 2014, pgs. 431.

Preface in Santoro,M. & Segre, C.A.M. in: **Complex Topics** in **Pediatrics**: **pediatric training** / editors Mario Santoro Junior and Conceigao Aparecida de Mattos Segre Sao Paulo, Editora Atheneu, 2015, pgs. 579.

Revelagoes: 2011-2015 Affonso Renato Meira Sao Paulo, Expressao & Arte Editora, 2016, pgs. 184.

Sixty years past: stories of a non-specialist doctor / Affonso Renato Meira, Sao Paulo, Scortecci, 2016, pgs. 178.

Legal and Ethical Aspects of Corrections in *Childhood and Adolescence* **in Plastic Surgery in Childhood and Adolescence** / editors Mario Santoro Junior and Juarez Avelar, Sao Paulo, Editora Atheneu in preparation.

Articles, lectures and courses.

He has published more than a hundred articles in scientific journals in Brazil, Argentina, Colombia, Ecuador, the United States of America, Portugal, Italy and England.

He has lectured in Brazil, Argentina, Colombia, Jamaica, Mexico, the United States of America, England, Lugoslavia, Peru, Scotland, Puerto Rico, Venezuela, Portugal, Spain, Azores and Turkey.

He has given courses at the Federal University of Mato Grosso do Sul, Grande Rio University, Federal University of Montes Claros, University of Western Santa Catarina, Sao Paulo School of Sociology and Politics, Latin American School of Bioethics, Sao Paulo Hospital Nursing School, Catholic University of Santos, Federal University of Maranhao, Institute for Economic and Social Development, University of Western São Paulo, University of the City of Sao Paulo, Kentucky University, Ataturk University and University of Sao Paulo.

He wrote articles, chronicles and commentaries in magazines and newspapers in the city of São Paulo.

Awards and honors received

Oscar Freire Award for Forensic Medicine and Criminology (1961)
Honorary host of the Royal Society for Public Health, London, England. (1969)
Fundacentro Award from the Occupational Medicine Foundation. (1998)
Honorary host of the Faculty of Medical Sciences and the Municipality of La Plata, Argentina (1989)
Vault of Brazilian Forensic Medicine at the XI Brazilian Congress of Forensic Medicine (1990)
Sao-Pauline Order of Perseverance (1994)
Gold Medal for outstanding service to the Hospital das Clinicas, Faculty of Medicine, University of Sao Paulo (1994)
Professor Emeritus of the Faculty of Medicine of the University of Sao Paulo.(2004)
Order of the Noble Knights of Sao Paulo of the Nove de Julho Battalion.(2004)
Diploma of Cultural Merit of the Brazilian Academy of Art, Culture and History.(2007)
Man of the Year in the Legislative Assembly of the State of São Paulo (2008)
ApparEnza Magazine's Man of Success (2013)
Awarded the Golden Jubilee of the Sovereign International Order of Sports Merit (2014)

Theses defended "Contribution to the study of the behavior of the maximum width and length of the head of white schoolchildren in the city of Sao Paulo."

Thesis presented to the Faculty of Dentistry of the University of Sao Paulo for the degree of Doctor. Chair of Preventive and Social Dentistry.

Defense on March 24, 1965, with a grade of 9.8.

Judging Panel of Professors:
Guilherme Oswaldo Arbenz;
Octavio Della Serra;
Milton Picosse;
Orlando Marques de Paiva;
Odorico Machado de Souza.

"Social Medical Study of the Contributing Factors to Conventional Business Aircraft Accidents between 1971 and 1975".

Thesis submitted to the Department of Forensic Medicine, Social and Occupational Medicine and Medical Deontology, USP Medical School, for the position of Full Professor.

Defense on October 18, 1976, passed with a 9.93 grade.

Judging Panel of Professors:
Armando Canger Rodrigues;
Guilherme Oswaldo Arbenz;
Edson da Silveira;
Milton Sejala Pauletto;
Jose Maria Marlet Pareta.

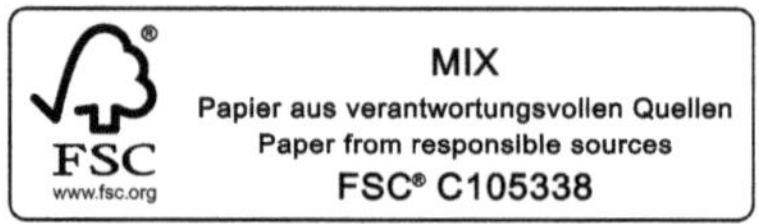

Printed by Books on Demand GmbH, Norderstedt / Germany